Healthy Profits
The 5 Elements of Strategic Wellness

By Sandra Larkin

Kathy Cash
Dr. Darren R. Weissman
Dori Babcock
Tara Zachgo, BS
Leslie Kahn
Merrilee Shopland, MA
Anne Ward
Bob Sandidge
Andrea H. Brockman, RN, DDS
Diana Stratigakis, MAPP
Billie Jo Hance, BS
Katy D. Quinn, RN, BSN
Janice Newman, SPHR, MHRM, CELS
Nicole Pfeffer Crombie
Jonathan Klane, M.S.Ed., CIH, CHMM, CET
Brian Leonard
Dr. Arien van der Merwe, MBChB, FRIPH, FRCAM
Retta Flagg
Patrice Rancour, MS, RN, CS
Kirsti A. Dyer, MD, MS
Rajiv Kumar
David Lazear
Devin Hakala, MS, LMFT
Lizzie Linton
Mr. Rooney
Sharon Glave Frazee, PhD
Ginger M. Barron-Brown, RPH
Sabrina Morgan-Graves, MD
Marcia Hamman, RN, BSN
Myra Wellingham, RN, MHA
Jeffery Davis, MBA

Healthy Profits
The 5 Elements of Strategic Wellness

ISBN 9824765-0-5

Copyright © 2009 by Sandra Larkin and Yellow Duck Press
Printed in the United States of America

Published by:
Yellow Duck Press
YellowDuckPress.com | HealthyProfitsBook.com

Creative, Graphic, Editorial and Production Services:
CreativeCore Media - .marketing.media.and.magic!
CreativeCore.com

All rights reserved. The purchase of this book entitles the purchaser to reproduce excerpts of the content for individual and small-group use. Chapters may be quoted or reproduced in their entirety on the condition that the full Authors credits and HealthyProfitsBook.com are credited and that the publisher is notified of each publication.

Beyond individual use, or as excepted, no form of this work may be reproduced, transmitted, posted, published, or recorded without permission from the publisher. Requests for permission should be addressed to Permissions@YellowDuckPress.com

Note: The information in this publication is for educational purposes only. The authors and publisher do not dispense medical advice or prescribe the use of any technique as treatment for physical, emotional, or medical issues without consultation with a qualified health care professional.

Table of Contents

Healthy Profits: Introduction..	7
Sandra Larkin My story...	12

Section 1: Physical Wellness

Introduction..	19
Physical Wellness: Personal Assessment...............................	21
The Mystery Revealed–WHY Wellness Works................... Kathy Cash	25
The Five Basics for Optimal Health: Discovering the Gift of Stress... Dr. Darren R. Weissman	31
Simple Tips for Eating Healthy.. Dori Babcock	39
Getting Active? Start SMART!... Tara Zachgo	43
Are We Sitting Comfortably? Then, Let's Begin................... Leslie Kahn	47

Section 2: Intellectual Wellness

Introduction..	53
Intellectual Wellness: Personal Assessment...........................	55
Your Wellness Vision: Turning Resolutions into Reality... Merrilee Shopland, MA	59
The Energizing Power of Focus.. Anne Ward and Bob Sandidge	63
Eliminating Dental Stress Leverages Wellness...................... Andrea H. Brockman, RN, DDS	69
Wellness Coaching: Partnering to Make Positive Changes...................................... Diana Stratigakis and Billie Jo Hance	75

Table of Contents

Section 3: Occupational Wellness

Introduction..	81
Occupational Wellness: Personal Assessment...................	83
Occupational Wellness..	87
Katy D. Quinn, RN, BSN	
Are You READY for Flexible Scheduling? The 8 hard questions you need to ask yourself!	91
Janice Newman	
Can that Strong Peppermint Candy Really Help Me to Focus? (The Answer: YES!).................	97
Nicole Pfeffer Crombie	
Combine Wellness with Workplace Safety and Health 12 Steps You Can Take to Increase Your Total Health!	103
Jonathan Klane, M.S.Ed., CIH, CHMM, CET	
Training your Business: The Proactive vs. Reactive Approach to a Safe Workplace.....................	109
Brian Leonard	

Section 4: Emotional Wellness

Introduction..	115
Emotional Wellness: Personal Assessment........................	117
Going for the Gold – Maintaining Work-Life Balance...............	121
Dr. Arien van der Merwe, MBChB, FRIPH, FRCAM	
To Err Is Human–To Forgive Is Healthy...........................	127
Retta Flagg	
Emotional Wellness: Keeping It Real and Keeping Your Cool When All Around You Others are Losing Theirs...............	131
Patrice Rancour, MS, RN, CS	

Table of Contents

Loss and the Workplace:
What to Do at Work When the World
Crashes in Around You.. 135
    Kirsti A. Dyer, MD, MS

Section 5: Social Wellness

Introduction... 145

Social Wellness: Personal Assessment... 148

Shape Up The Nation: Using Our Social Networks
To Promote Wellness... 151
    Rajiv Kumar

Whole Brain Thinking and Planning... 155
    David Lazear

The Poison of Workplace Gossip... 163
    Devin Hakala, MS, LMFT

Boundaries on the Clock: Stories to Live By................................ 167
    Lizzie Linton

Being Social and Productive... 171
    Mr. Rooney

Section 6: Putting It All Together

Introduction... 177

Learning by Example: Leveraging Clinicians at the
Worksite for Better Health and Wellness..................................... 179
    Sharon Glave Frazee, PhD, Ginger M. Barron-Brown,
    RPH, Sabrina Morgan-Graves, MD, Marcia Hamman,
    RN, BSN, Myra Wellingham, RN, MHA, and Jeffery
    Davis, MBA

Putting It All Together:
Whole Person Strategic Wellness.. 185
    Sandra Larkin

"The concept of total wellness recognizes that our every thought, word, and behavior affects our greater health and well-being. And we, in turn, are affected not only emotionally but also physically and spiritually."
  ~ Greg Anderson, founder of
  The American Wellness Project

Introduction

Congratulations on taking a well deserved big giant leap towards health and wellness. Right now, you may be in either one of two stages in your health journey. Are you beginning a personal transformation, moving one step closer to improved health? Or, are you a seasoned health veteran looking for more information to maintain or reach new health levels? Regardless of where you begin or where you end up, it's the journey combined with knowledge that creates the "stick to it" glue in reaching the why of our goals. Here is a formula to help make the journey interesting and successful.

Personal Desire (The Why) +
    Increased Health Knowledge (The How) +
        Action Plan (The When) =
            Successful Health Journey

When I began my professional career in the early 1980's, the concept of wellness in the workplace was in its infancy. According to James William Miller in *Wellness: The History and Development of a Concept,* "By the late 1970s, the wellness movement was well under way in the United States. Some businesses were beginning to offer workplace wellness programs." Armed with my passion for staying healthy, I sought to develop my own wellness program. At that time, I had no clue that what I designed and implemented on a personal level would be considered a wellness program as we know it today.

I included activities that would keep me fit in five strategic elements of wellness: physical, intellectual, social, occupational, and emotional. I read self help books, attended free hospital seminars, tried healthy recipes and healthy lifestyle suggestions. This was all in an effort to become and stay healthy at all moments in my life. I was not looking at the magazines and media to be my guide. I had other goals that were important and wanted to incorporate these into a total healthy lifestyle for the long haul.

Introduction

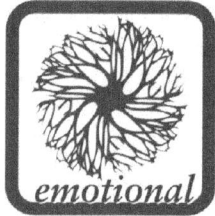
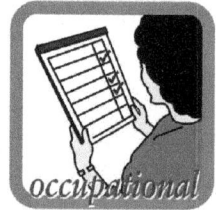
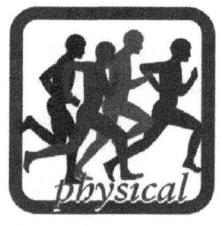

5 Elements of Strategic Wellness

So why the five elements of strategic wellness? Because a variety of wellness activities keeps our whole person on a healthy even keel. We can be physically healthy but socially in poor health if we don't know how to connect with our co-workers on a daily basis. We can be an intellectual genius at our job but emotionally incapable of working out conflict in the workplace and build strong teams. Health is not all physical—it's not all of any one of the five strategic areas. It is a unique, continual learning and dynamic balancing act between all five elements: physical, emotional, intellectual, social, and occupational. Along the way, we become healthy and prosperous as we see what learning new skills does for our self-esteem, confidence, and internal profits. Our organizations benefit, as we become our best, reach goals for our department, and increase revenue for our organization.

The thirty-one wellness experts in this book will help you gain the knowledge to make the journey interesting in each of the five strategic elements. These professionals have hundreds of years of combined experience serving global populations, helping to maintain and improve health and well-being. In addition, most of these specialists are already published authors and well known health bloggers in the wellness community. Their expertise can help you move one step closer to your personal health goals.

From CEO's to nurses, their education and accreditation reaches into the heart of the wellness profession. Accomplished and credible, they are dedicated to and passionate about helping you and your organization reach your health and wellness goals. Daily, they see the consequences of poor health choices and celebrate the accomplishments of health success. Their knowledge extends beyond the bounds of their practices into the wellness community with integrity and impact. Now it extends to you!

Wellness In The Workplace: The Why?

The average American spends well over 40 hours working per week. Increased demands from global competition, fewer resources and tighter deadlines mean that work consumes a vast majority of our days. Over an extended period of time, this leads to feeling overworked, overwhelmed, stressed, negative, and unproductive.

How about that commute? The Gallup Organization annual Work and Education survey from 2007 found that "American workers report spending an average of 46 minutes commuting to and from work in a typical day."[1] This survey also showed that "The vast majority of workers say their commute is not that stressful, but workers who travel at least an hour each day are much more likely than those who travel less than that to say their commute is stressful."

And then there's what we do when we're not working that also asks us for our time in polite and not so polite ways. The Bureau of Labor Statistics has compiled a list of personal care activities that take our time on a daily basis. By the way, don't forget to include the holidays and special event party planning.

---

[1] http://www.gallup.com/poll/28504/Workers-Average-Commute-RoundTrip-Minutes-Typical-Day.aspx

Introduction

Personal care activities [2]

- Sleeping
- Eating and drinking
- Household activities
- Housework
- Food preparation and cleanup
- Lawn and garden care
- Household management
- Purchasing goods and services
- Consumer goods purchases
- Professional and personal care services
- Caring for and helping household
- Members
- Children
- Caring for and helping non-household
- Members
- Adults
- Working
- Work-related activities
- Educational Activities
- Attending class
- Homework and research
- Organizational, civic, and religious activities
- Religious and spiritual activities
- Volunteering (Organizational and civic activities)
- Leisure and sports
- Socializing and communicating
- Watching Television
- Participating in sports, exercise, and recreation
- Telephone calls, mail, and e-mail

---

[2] List compiled from Bureau of Labor Statistics
http://www.bls.gov/news.release/atus.t08.htm

Other activities

Between work, commute, and personal responsibilities, where does personal health and fitness fit into the mix on a daily, weekly, or monthly basis? It stands to reason that if we are spending more time at work then why not practice wellness at the worksite to keep healthy?

The number of employers implementing specific wellness programs increased three times from 2007 to 2008. In 2008, for example, the top five wellness programs implemented were promoting physical activity (68% vs. 19% in 2007); disease management programs (60% vs. 18%); health risk appraisals (48% vs. 14%); biometric screening (47% vs. 12%); and telephonic health care coaching (45% vs. 14%) according to Aon Consulting's *2008 Benefits and Talent Survey.* [3]

Ok, here it comes! The response, "I don't have time to take a lunch—how can I take time to exercise or attend other wellness program events?" The answer is—drum roll please—step away from the desk. If you are thinking that you have no time, you're right. It's a conscious and deliberate choice to put one hour of the day towards an activity that will make you healthy and productive. For example, lunch. Try walking, attending a wellness event at work, chilling out, or choosing healthy foods and portions throughout the day. Adelle Davis, a noted nutritionist, is quoted, "As I see it, every day you do one of two things: build health or produce disease in yourself."

The choice is yours.

---

[3] http://www.ccibenefitsolutions.com/content/HRinsider/MayHRinsider08.html

Introduction

Sandra Larkin My story

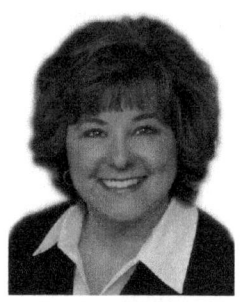

"I need to be honest; I think you have a brain tumor. I'm sending you for an MRI. The massive headaches and vision loss you are experiencing are indications that there may be a brain tumor present."

Sitting on the physician's exam table in June of 2004, I tried to take in the initial diagnosis. I wasn't thinking about the company I worked for in terms of their goals, projects, my direct reports or how much work I left at the office. All I was thinking was, "How did I get here?" A flood of emotion as well as anger filled my thoughts. I took pride each day in making small consistent changes towards health. How could this happen to me?

Days after the MRI was performed, I was back in the doctor's office sitting on the same exam table waiting for him to enter the room. Would it be good news or bad? What would happen to my family? Is this going to hurt? Am I going to die?

Ultimately, what he would tell me would change the course of my life. As my doctor entered the room, I examined his face. His expression was not stressed. His brow wasn't furrowed but he also wasn't smiling. He began, "I'm happy to report you don't have a brain tumor. All of your symptoms are caused from a toxic stress combination. You will need to quit your job tomorrow in order to live to see your daughter graduate from high school. If stress is producing these types of symptoms on the outside, what's it doing to the inside of your body? This includes your heart, arteries and internal organs. You need to make drastic changes, immediately, to live."

What? Quit my job? That's crazy. I love my job. My boss is a great mentor. I enjoy the people I work with and can manage just fine. So what if I have a few headaches and can't see sometimes? Also, the extreme acid reflux I have been dealing with is under control on prescription medication. Hey, that's why they make prescription drugs. So what if my company does not offer any type of wellness program. I guess I should be glad that I have a job and shouldn't look to them for help in health and wellness. Intense job stress? I guess that's the price we pay. It doesn't matter that I'm not

Healthy Profits

getting any management relief from project conflicts that include people conflict too. Hit or miss professional training is fine with me. I don't have time, anyway. What's he talking about when he says a "toxic stress combination"?

Let's take a look at <u>my typical day.</u>

- Wake up at 3:30 a.m. to exercise and meditate
- Get ready for work and leave by 6:30 a.m.
- Drive 37 miles one way in Chicago traffic
- Work a ten hour day which includes about four to six hours of meetings
- Walk at lunch time then graze on a salad all afternoon
- Go to the convenience store in the building at 3:00 p.m. with a few of my colleagues for chocolate and junk food
- Drive 37 miles back home in the same Chicago traffic
- Make dinner and take care of my family while I'm exhausted
- Go to bed by 10:00 p.m. or sometimes at 7:00 p.m.

Humm... is this the toxic stress combination he was talking about?

Does it include ...
- Grocery shopping
- Running errands
- Paying bills
- Cleaning
- Attending school events
- Homework
- Socializing with friends
- Trying to maintain a marriage relationship
- Traveling for business
- Maintaining the household chores with my husband
- Working out solutions to extended family personal and health issues 500 miles away on a daily basis

Introduction

What happened to my own personal wellness plan I had in place? I thought it was working. I'll just ignore what the physician ordered and see what happens next. This can't be as out of control as it appears.

It took an additional six months of being extremely sick to make the decision to resign my company position. In February of 2005, my body and mind could no longer function. The fact remained that I was not getting better but maintaining failing health. In addition, the stress from the job was too much for me to handle.

<u>What did I gain by making the decision to resign and right size my health?</u>

I gained a feeling of loss and triumph but not at the same time. Loss from a job I loved and health gained within three months of my resignation. Right after I resigned, I signed up for a three month daily boot camp at my fitness club. I was GI Jane—it was extremely intense both physically and mentally. Mentally, it cleared my mind of the intensity with which I was pursuing life and career. It removed me from a job situation that was no longer healthy for me and was not negotiable. Daily, I would apply heat to some areas of my body and ice to others.

At the end of the three months, my stress symptoms were gone. I lost two dress sizes and my clinical readings where normal. Then, I began the healing process with my family members who also took a direct hit from my stress.

What did my company lose in the process?

My company lost ....

- An eight-year, mid-level manager who was passionate about the job, the company, its people and customers
- A 20 year corporate veteran with a broad range of expertise
- A valuable and experienced organizational knowledge base which walked right out the door on February 11, 2005
- A person who was generally liked in the workplace as evidenced by current long term lasting work relationships after the resignation

- A woman who had a passion and dream for the company, then right sized it into a thriving business of her own

We can wonder if the company lost the respect and confidence of other employees as they watched this situation unfold. Was their public image tarnished as employees talked in outside private circles about this situation and what would happen to them if the same events occurred? Was there an underlying current of "what if's" and lack of respect for senior management at the water cooler? Could someone have done something in the company? I guess we'll never know.

Keep in mind that my same situation is playing out throughout the world of work daily. Change the place of business and the employee name and you have a "toxic stress combination" that can affect organizational revenue, profit, goal attainment, customer satisfaction, and public image.

In the end, I've moved on to a better place physically, emotionally, intellectually, occupationally and socially. That which was life threatening became life changing. I have used this disadvantage to the advantage of others and myself by moving into the workplace wellness arena for the betterment not only of employers but directly helping employees as well.

Sitting on one side of the cubicle—and the other side of the boardroom table—brings a unique perspective on wellness in the workplace. We don't need to lose the company expertise or invest our total profit margin into a wellness program. Organizations can and should put some well care into the workplace for people to thrive and survive, at the same time helping to create healthy profits in people and, ultimately, in the bottom line.

Sandra Larkin, CWPM is uniquely qualified to provide objective direction, creativity and strategic direction in planning and delivering wellness initiatives to achieve profit-focused objectives. She maintains key partnerships in her global strategic network of wellness professionals that provide her client base with a distinct competitive advantage. Sandra is a national motivational speaker and trainer on health and wellness in the workplace. sandra@sandralarkin.com   www.SandraLarkin.com

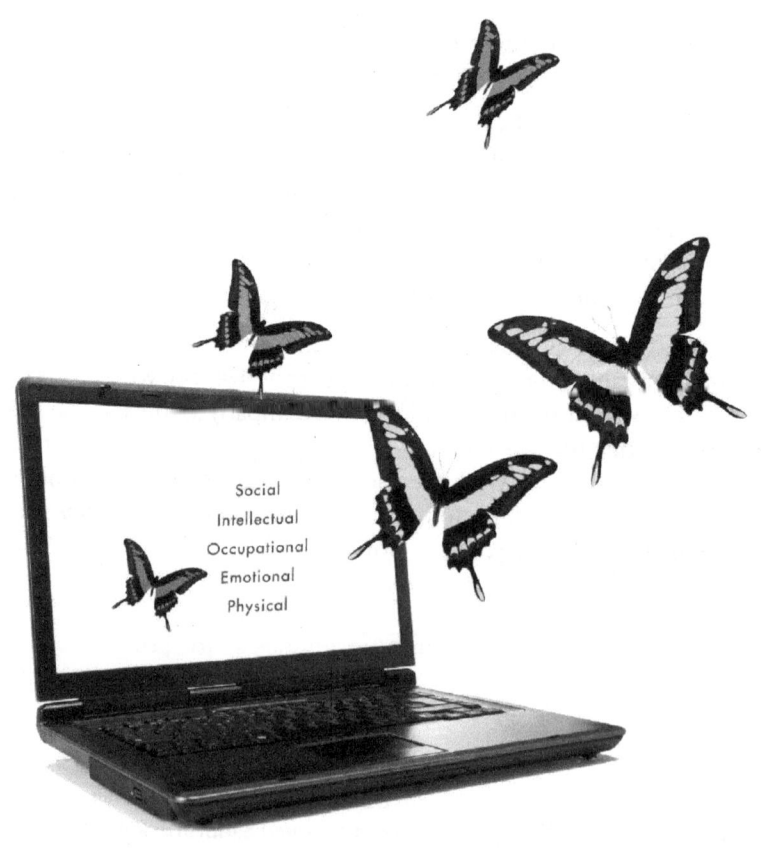

Section 1: Physical Wellness

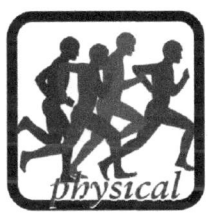

"Over the years I have developed a picture of what a human being living humanely is like. She is a person who understands, values and develops her body, finding it beautiful and useful; a person who is real and is willing to take risks, to be creative, to manifest competence, to change when the situation calls for it, and to find ways to accommodate to what is new and different, keeping that part of the old that is still useful and discarding what is not.
~ *Virginia Satir*

Section 1: Physical Wellness

Introduction

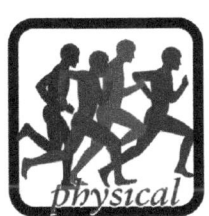

Physical Wellness encourages proper nutrition, regular physical activities, and health care. It seeks healthy alternatives in place of dependence on tobacco, alcohol, or other drugs. It reduces the number of sick days over the long and short term of an associate's career. Physical wellness is achieved by expanding the knowledge needed to live a healthy lifestyle, good nutrition, and physical activities that reduce stress. It also assists in the total well-being of the body as flexibility, strength, and cardiovascular health are improved. It encourages preventive measures and monitoring of ones health numbers such as blood pressure, cholesterol, and weight.

Characteristics of Physical Wellness:

- Awareness of behaviors that are detrimental to health (illegal drug use, smoking, excessive alcohol use, food choices)
- Knowledge in the areas of overall health risk and assessment
- Education about balanced nutrition including quantity and quality of food sources
- Practice of physical fitness to maintain overall physical health and increase health-related benefits
- Avoidance of environmental issues that contribute to an unhealthy lifestyle (second-hand smoke, pollutants, nonuse of seat belts or sunscreen)
- Maintenance of adequate sleep levels

Physical wellness encompasses respect for our own body type and uniqueness. We begin to engage in actions that move us toward acquiring a higher level of health. Our enhanced physical health steers us away from harmful behaviors and habits while we focus on total fitness. We begin to feel comfortable with a strong body and treat it with respect.

The Need for Physical Wellness

Did you know that ...

Americans are fighting the battle of their lives—the battle against obesity—and have grown larger and larger over the past century. Currently, we are reaching obesity levels at epidemic proportions. A contributing factor to America's rapid weight gain is the food we eat.

The following statistics shed light on how we approach food in America today:

- The typical American now consumes three hamburgers and four orders of French fries every week.
- Americans now spend more money on fast food than on higher education, personal computers, computer software, or new cars.
- In 1999, of the 30 fastest growing US franchises, 12 were fast food—only three were nutrition and fitness.

Source: Fast Food Nation by Eric Schlosser

Physical Wellness Experts

In this section, we'll learn "Why Wellness Works" from **Kathy Cash**. We begin to migrate through the mystery of wellness and learn anti-aging tips.

Next, discover the "Five Basics for Optimal Health" with **Dr. Darren Weissman**. How do water, food, rest, exercise, and owning your own power provide us with a foundation for working with stress?

In addition, **Dori Babcock** gets down to basics with "Simple Tips For Healthy Eating." Dori outlines easy methods to increase your nutritional intake during the course of a day.

Healthy Profits

With increased nutrition comes activity. **Tara Zachgo** helps us look at ways to increase exercise with activities we love with "Getting Active? Start Smart."

Once we're back at our desks, **Leslie Kahn** details prevention of body stress by outlining how to sit comfortably plus other desk related challenges such as eyestrain and telephone neck.

Let's begin.

Physical Wellness: Personal Assessment

Read the questions and rate yourself from 0 (low level) to 5 (high level) of achievement. Determine the total number for each rating and compare it to the answer key below. This determines where your physical wellness stands today. Take the test again in 30 days to check your progress on improving physical wellness. Remember, improvement in any area is *positive action in motion*.

1. I exercise at least three times per week for 30 minutes or more.

    5   4   3   2   1   0

2. I walk a minimum of 10,000 steps per day.

    5   4   3   2   1   0

3. I consume at least 80-90% of my weekly food in a nutritious way.

    5   4   3   2   1   0

4. I change up my exercise routine to challenge my body and remove boredom.

    5   4   3   2   1   0

5. I maintain regular health appointments, screenings and vaccinations.

    5   4   3   2   1   0

Physical Wellness

6. I eat breakfast every day.

       5   4   3   2   1   0

7. I generally have good feelings about my body image.

       5   4   3   2   1   0

8. I am aware of my health numbers like weight, blood pressure, and cholesterol.

       5   4   3   2   1   0

9. I seek to "get healthy" versus have a specific body size, shape, or weight number.

       5   4   3   2   1   0

10. I am a continual learner of health-related information and how to stay healthy.

        5   4   3   2   1   0

Answer Key: If you answered,

    Mostly 5's you have an excellent level of physical wellness. Continue stretching your comfort zone and finding ways to gain greater benefits of being physically fit. Consider teaching others how they can reach their physical wellness goals.

    Mostly 4's you have a high level of physical wellness. Consider finding innovative ways to make your 4's turn to 5's. This can be fun and exciting.

    Mostly 3's you have a reasonable level of physical wellness. With a greater attempt and laser focus, you become the model of what it takes to get where you want to be.

    Mostly 2's you're at a good starting point of physical wellness. Allow yourself to begin again, set goals and go for it!

Mostly 1's it's time for an upgrade. You have what it takes. Make yourself a priority. Wellness is important to thrive and survive in todays fast pace world.

Mostly 0's choose one area of physical wellness to improve upon each month. Seek a buddy to help you find ways to reach your goal, hold you accountable and be your cheerleader. You're worth the investment!

"The power of love to change bodies is legendary, built into folklore, common sense, and everyday experience. Love moves the flesh, it pushes matter around.... Throughout history, 'tender loving care' has uniformly been recognized as a valuable element in healing."

~ Larry Dossey

The Mystery Revealed
WHY Wellness Works

Kathy Cash

Were you a wellness holdout? You know, one of those people who said, "I'm going to die of something, so why worry?" As you got older, maybe you began to realize dying isn't the only consequence of unhealthy behaviors... that years of disability and poor health could lay ahead for you because of poor choices? If so, I have good news. It's not too late to change that future, regardless of your age.

I started working in health promotion (or wellness) 30 years ago. The industry was in its infancy then. Often recommendations grew from years of simply watching people and noticing links between lifestyle and what ultimately made them sick.

We knew people who smoked, abused alcohol, didn't exercise, and ate mostly junk food often suffered from illnesses such as heart disease, strokes, cancers, and diabetes. But we also knew that people who exercised; ate lots of fruits, veggies, and lean meats; and managed life stresses tended to live longer and experience fewer diseases and conditions associated with old age.

What we didn't know (then) was "why" this was true. There were certainly many theories but surprisingly little hard science. As a result, many people, including some in the medical profession, were slow to embrace wellness programs and recommendations.

As time went by, skepticism waned. Scientific research began proving what we knew intuitively. Anti-aging medicine grew as a specialized field. A relative newcomer in the field of medicine, "anti-aging" refers to any activity that slows, prevents, or even reverses aging.

To understand "anti"-aging, you must first understand aging. I'll never forget going to a 20-year high school reunion. We were surrounded by classmates. They were all the same age, yet some looked old enough to be their friends' parents. Others seemed to have barely aged since graduation. How could people age so differently? That question lies at the heart of aging research.

Obviously, aging is the act of growing older, when our abilities begin to decline and battles with disease and poor health become more common. How quickly (or slowly) we experience these changes depends on a combination of genes, environment, and lifestyle. Anti-aging medicine seeks to modify these factors in your favor... *to keep you as young as possible, as long as possible.*

Among the most potent weapons in today's "anti-aging" arsenal are key body hormones. What are hormones? Basically, hormones tell cells what to do.

The longer explanation... and I promise it won't be too technical... is that hormones are chemicals released by cells in one part of the body that affect what cells do in other parts of the body. Cells responding to a hormone's "message" do so because they produce a specific molecule (or receptor) on their surface. Think of these "receptors" as a lock on the cell door. Only the right hormone has the key to unlock the door and deliver its message. All other hormones will be rejected by the cell. There are a great many hormones and each has a different message to deliver.

It's generally believed that hormone levels decrease with age. Insufficient quantities of a hormone means target cells don't get instructions to do their jobs. This leads to disease and premature aging.

The question now being asked is how much does lifestyle affect the extent of this hormone decline? We do know that when an aging body's hormones are brought back to more youthful levels, there is a powerful rejuvenating effect. The person feels, acts, and looks younger.

While these potent (and often expensive) hormones can be replaced artificially by an appropriately certified physician, that application is not the purpose of this article. Instead, let's focus on how you can naturally increase production of important hormones through healthier lifestyles.

Human Growth Hormone – The Master Hormone

One of the most important hormones is Human Growth Hormone (HGH). Originally known for helping children grow tall, for many years it was thought that HGH had no real benefits to fully-grown humans. Thanks to anti-aging medicine, we know that maintaining youthful HGH levels has many proven benefits for aging adults:

- Healthier and younger looking skin
- Faster healing and reduced infections after injury or surgery
- Decreased total body fat
- Increased lean muscle mass
- Increased bone mineral density
- Improved cholesterol blood levels
- Improved libido
- Better stamina and endurance during exercise
- Quicker recovery time between workouts
- Improved mood, coping skills, and overall well-being
- Improved energy levels

Other hormones support HGH in slowing the aging process. Some of the additional benefits of this hormone team are to improve brain function, reduce risks for cardiovascular disease, and improve immunity.

Look again at the above list. When people complain about the more common negative signs of aging, the symptoms they often describe are the symptoms of LOW levels of HGH and supporting hormones. Logically, raising these key hormones should help improve signs of early aging.

Lifestyle and Hormone Production

Many lifestyle issues fall under the umbrella of wellness. But most professionals agree physical activity, avoiding tobacco and other risky substances; stress management, proper nutrition, and maintaining an ideal weight are the key behaviors influencing good health.

Here's where it gets exciting. Look at the impact lifestyle has on HGH levels:

- Fitness – Regular aerobic and anaerobic activity stimulates HGH production
- Smoking, drug abuse, and overuse of alcohol – Slows HGH production
- High quality nutritious foods and avoiding overeating – Enhances HGH production
- Stress – Chronic unrelieved stress slows HGH production
- Sleep – High quality sleep encourages HGH production
- Obesity – Slows HGH production and when HGH levels are raised, efforts at weight loss are more successful

Get the picture? Healthy lifestyles help keep HGH levels up and poor lifestyles decrease ideal levels of HGH.

The Anti-Aging Wellness Program

As I mentioned, anti-aging physicians can replace low levels of HGH, and in diagnosed deficiencies, it can be very beneficial. But wouldn't it make more sense... and be cheaper... to simply adopt behaviors that help your body produce ideal amounts of HGH on its own?

- Don't use tobacco... or quit
- If you drink alcohol, do so only in moderation... one or two glasses a day
- Eat a diet rich in antioxidants such as vitamins C, E, and beta carotene
- Eat frequent small meals throughout the day rather than a few big ones
- Reduce intake of saturated fats and increase intake of Omega-3 oils
- Eat high quality, lean proteins

- Drink plenty of filtered water and other non-caffeinated liquids
- Daily exercise should be a combination of aerobic and anaerobic activities (Note: It's OK to alternate which days you do a particular type of exercise, as long as you get all types in each week)
- Practice effective stress management techniques, such as meditation and yoga
- Develop life skills to deal with change and stress (Examples: anger management, communication, assertiveness, self-esteem)
- Get periodic age-, risk-, gender-specific physical examinations
- Evaluate and modify your environment for sources of toxins
- Do everything possible to get the best quality sleep (Note: If you have been told you snore... a lot... get evaluated for sleep apnea)
- Never stop learning – Keep the brain active
- Get evaluated for other hormone deficiencies – Discuss hormonal treatment of menopause and andropause (male "menopause") with your health care provider (Another concern: An under-active thyroid is one of the most under-diagnosed problems of older adults)

To Supplement or Not to Supplement

Think of nutrition supplements as "health insurance." Meeting nutritional needs becomes more difficult with age. Digestion and nutrient absorption become less efficient. Vitamin and mineral deficiencies are often misdiagnosed as serious illnesses in seniors. These potential problems can be greatly reduced with the aid of nutritional supplements.

Nutrition "purists" will tell you that nutrition supplements aren't necessary. In a perfect world I would agree with them, but this isn't a perfect world. We eat a lot of stuff, but it's the wrong stuff. Our lives are fast-paced. Getting the quality of food we need is challenging. Even the notoriously cautious American Medical

The Mystery Revealed–Why Wellness Works

Association endorses taking a daily multivitamin. Talk to your doctor or a nutritionist about other supplements that might be appropriate for your unique needs.

It's possible you don't need supplements, but isn't it worth the investment of a few extra cents a day to provide your body with those additional nutrients... just in case?

The Real Secret

Now that you have a plan for staying healthy and vital, what are you going to do with those vibrant golden years? Studies of healthy, happy seniors show a direct link between positive attitudes and aging. Don't obsess over the little things. Laugh off the occasional "senior moment." Don't allow regrets to rule your life. Learn from mistakes if you can, but ultimately, just move on. Life is about growing and changing. Spend your life having the time of your life. Preserve your youthful sense of curiosity and wonder and you will preserve your youth as well.

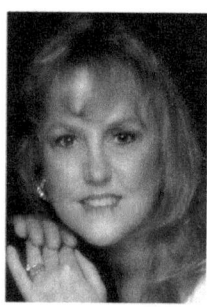

Kathy Cash, RN, CHPD, is a retired Lieutenant Colonel. One of the Air Force's top Health Promotion Administrators, Kathy went on to design the first Department of Defense prevention program for a Fortune 500 HMO. Now a freelance health/wellness writer and consultant, Kathy lives in Tennessee with husband, Grady.
cashk@comcast.net.

The Five Basics for Optimal Health: Discovering the Gift of Stress

Dr. Darren R. Weissman

Time Magazine recently reported that stress-related insurance claims, which include job burnout and depression, are now the fastest growing disability category. The situation is made worse, the magazine noted, because people tend to cope with chronic stress by watching television, skipping exercise, and forgoing healthy foods.

We all know that stress cannot be avoided. Everyone is always experiencing some type of stress, even while sleeping. But stress is not entirely undesirable—think about the stress of a successful work venture, an exhilarating experience, or of being in love. Now think about the stress caused by divorce, by being passed over for a promotion, or by receiving a traffic ticket. The stress reaction, depending upon the circumstances and the state of the body during the experience, is actually a gift. Stress is the language that your body and life use to help you reconnect to the power you possess to take responsibility for all aspects of your life.

Dr. Hans Selye was the physiologist whose observations of patients while in medical school led him to borrow the word "stress" from physicists and apply it to the biology of the human body. In the beginning, skeptics ridiculed Selye's assertions that stress was related to major illness, such as heart disease and cancer. It took more than 40 years of exhaustive research and impeccable methodology before Dr. Selye's findings led to the establishment of an entirely new medical field—the study of biological stress and its effects.

Because of Dr. Selye's painstaking efforts, the word "stress" is now a part of the world's lexicon. Soon after, stress, and stress-related disorders became the buzz of the latter 20th century work world, especially in the wake of a technological revolution that required employees to be able to both multi-task and perform multi-purpose functions in all aspects of their lives.

The Five Basics for Optimal Health:
Discovering the Gift of Stress

While the world has focused on the causes of stress, few noted one of Dr. Selye's most important observations during his research: He noticed that when patients experiencing high levels of stress were advised by their doctors to rest and eat easily digestible food—and they followed those directions—their health greatly improved.

Today, the impact of diet and rest, along with other key elements of a healthy lifestyle, are still under-valued despite the growing body of evidence that lifestyle is a key component of total well-being. I would like to recommend concrete ways you can mitigate, as well as understand, the empowering potential of stress: The Five Basics of Optimal Health.

Before I explain in detail The Five Basics, I am providing a stress assessment tool. Rather than focusing on the causes of stress, it focuses on preventing the ravaging effects of stress, by helping you create balance in both your body and life through maintaining the proper quantity, quality, and frequency of The Five Basics of Optimal Health—Water, Food, Rest, Exercise, and Own Your Power.

Stress Assessment

1. I drink one quart of quality water (not tap) for every 50 pounds of body weight daily.

    Yes_____   No_____

2. I drink an equal amount of water for every cup of coffee, tea, juice, soda, energy drink, or diet drink.

    Yes_____   No_____

3. I eat at least six to eight small meals every day.

    Yes_____   No_____

4. For snacks, I eat fruit or a helping of raw nuts.

    Yes_____   No_____

5. I do not eat refined sugar or white flour products.

    Yes_____   No_____

6. I sleep an average of seven or eight hours every night.

    Yes_____   No_____

7. I sleep soundly throughout the night, and wake up well rested.

    Yes_____   No_____

8. I exercise at least 30 minutes daily.

    Yes_____   No_____

9. I am passionate about what I do for a living.

    Yes_____   No_____

10. I am able to express feelings easily and clearly.

    Yes_____   No_____

Score:

9–10 "Yes" answers
You make self-care a priority and are tuned into your limitless potential to "go with the flow" in every situation. You are optimally empowered to handle any stressful situation.

6–8 "Yes" answers
You are aware of the importance of being pro-active about your health, and are somewhat in tune with the connection between your lifestyle and your ability to handle whatever hand life deals you.

5 or fewer "Yes" answers
You need a tune-up—a reminder that there is a "cause and effect" relationship between a health-affirming lifestyle and being able to positively respond to the daily stresses of life.

*The Five Basics for Optimal Health:
Discovering the Gift of Stress*

Here is why these issues are critical to the body's ability to adapt and positively respond to stress:

Water

Your body is composed of 75 percent water and 25 percent solid matter. Brain tissue is 85 percent water; blood is 82 percent; and the lungs are nearly 90 percent. The body is like a sponge: it's made up of trillions of cells that absorb and hold water. According to the late Dr. F. Batmanghelidj, a medical doctor and the author of the book, <u>Your Body's Many Cries for Water</u>, the need for water is an essential part of human evolution. Water is the primary conductor of electricity that operates all of the body's major functions—thinking, circulation, breathing, and elimination—and each one is dependent upon water to function optimally.

Dehydration affects blood pressure, blood sugar metabolism, digestion, and kidney function, as well as the ability to think clearly. Coffee, sugar-filled coffee drinks, regular and diet soda, herbal and black tea, sports drinks, energy drinks, and concentrated juices all contribute to dehydration, especially if the person does not drink an equal amount of water for every one of those beverages consumed.

The ability to positively handle stress can best be achieved and maintained when we drink one quart (32 ounces) of quality, filtered water for every 50 pounds of body weight, rounding up to the highest quart. For example, a 180 pound person would need to drink four quarts, or 128 ounces, of water on a daily basis. As noted earlier, for every non-water beverage that is consumed, you should consume an equal additional amount of water.

Food

Sugar is extremely addictive, has no nutritional value, is high in calories, and prompts the body to enter a degenerative state because it leads to insulin sensitivity. Most eating programs today are too high in simple carbohydrates (sugar): enriched and whole-grain refined flour (bread, donuts, muffins, and crackers); pasta, rice, concentrated sweeteners (sugar, fructose, and honey), ice cream—even ketchup. Carbohydrates, simple and complex, ultimately break down into simple sugars. Digested and assimilated rapidly by the body, they can provide quick, short-term energy, raise the blood-sugar levels and stimulate the production of insulin. But eating too many carbohydrates or not enough protein causes the body to become imbalanced. This imbalance can manifest as a number of symptoms, including poor stress response, mood swings, poor concentration, headaches, sugar cravings, depression, allergies, hyperactivity, memory loss, spaciness, rashes, chronic fatigue, inflammation of the joints and muscles, frequent colds, and learning disabilities.

The only way to control that balance is through food selection—choosing foods that are high in protein (eggs, meat, raw nuts), low in simple carbohydrates (no processed foods), and contain healthy fat. By eating six to eight small meals per day comprised of high-quality foods, in a ratio that includes 80 percent green (alkaline) food, as well as drinking water, you can help the body combat the negative aspects of stress.

Rest

There's a direct link between the quality of your rest and the ability to positively respond to stressful situations. Far too many people suffer from insomnia. The causes include an eating program that's too high in sugar and refined carbohydrates, dehydration, physical or emotional trauma, and not getting enough exercise.

Sleep deprivation not only affects the body's immune system, it can speed up the aging process and the onset of metabolic or hormonal imbalances. In addition to fatigue, some of the effects of a lack of sleep include weight gain, irritability, blurred vision, slurring of speech, short-term memory lapses, an inability to concentrate, and hallucinations.

Keep in mind that the amount of rest necessary is impacted by the state of health, level of stress, and age. Any posture held for an extended period of time, such as hunching over a computer keyboard or bending the neck to read, also will impact your ability to sleep.

Posture, as well as the quantity and quality of rest, plays a major role in overall well-being. The healthiest posture for sleeping is on either side or your back. On average, you should get between seven and nine hours of sleep per night—children need more. Making sure you receive quality rest and relaxation is the most

The Five Basics for Optimal Health:
Discovering the Gift of Stress

significant step you can take to reduce the stress of modern living so that you can be healthier and happier.

Exercise

Most of us are obsessed with our weight instead of being focused on our health. Unfortunately, despite the millions of dollars earned by the makers of lose-weight-quick supplements, there isn't a single item on the market that turns an obese body into a healthy, stress-resistant one. Research has found that everyone can benefit from regular physical activity, and physical decline associated with aging can even be reversed through exercise.

Fitness is multifaceted, so you need a program that addresses the issue from all angles. Recent studies have shown that 30-60 minutes of daily exercise improves your body's ability to handle stress; use insulin and metabolize food; maintain a healthy weight; increase energy levels and mental clarity; develop healthy bones, muscles and joints; be stronger; improve balance; reduce feelings of depression and anxiety; and heighten self esteem.

Begin with something as simple as breathing exercises that include mild muscle contraction-relaxation sequences to help you connect with your body. You also can walk, run, engage in weight training, Yoga, Pilates, or Tai chi.

Own Your Power

When you don't express your emotions authentically, you force your body to find another language to communicate them. Notice, for example, when you find someone difficult to deal with, that person literally becomes "a pain in the neck." Or think about the times when you have had a "gut reaction" to a person or event. This "body language" can also be a pain, organ dysfunction, imbalanced sugar metabolism, or reveal itself as numerous other symptoms associated with the mind-body-spirit connection. Denying your intuitive feelings causes the body to speak out—the longer you internalize your feelings, the louder it will yell.

Owning your power means to embrace all aspects of life—especially the stressful experiences—with passion, conviction, and courage. It means embracing change and the emotions associated with that change. There are many ways to connect with your feelings—exercise, meditation, journaling, writing poetry, forgiveness, music, dancing, and painting. But ultimately, it comes down to embracing all aspects of your life with the attitude of gratitude.

The Attitude of Gratitude is the greatest stress resistor

The attitude you have toward any experience is a choice. At any given moment, you can always view the cup as being half full or half empty, but the most courageous way to move through life is by choosing to find the good in every instant. Rather than surrendering to the emotions of negativity and despair, consciously and creatively embrace life with the attitude of gratitude. Accepting challenges as opportunities immediately transforms each situation into a chance to develop your higher self. The act of expressing appreciation, such as saying thank you, symbolizes the value an experience has had for you. The attitude of gratitude expands your view of an experience beyond the "self" to an infinite perspective of possibilities and potential. By embracing all stressful situations with the gratitude, you'll discover the real value and meaning of your life. Gratitude is the ultimate weapon against stress.

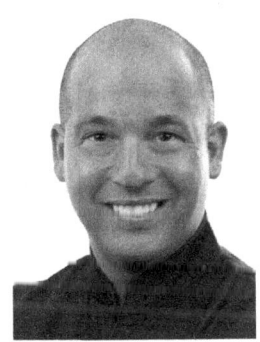

Dr. Darren R. Weissman, is the author of The Power of Infinite Love & Gratitude, an internationally renowned teacher and speaker, and the developer of The LifeLine Technique™. The LifeLine Technique™ is an advanced holistic system that builds upon the work of Louise L. Hay, Dr. Bruce Lipton, Gregg Braden, and Dr. Masaru Emoto, fusing science and spirit by harmonizing emotions buried within the subconscious mind
www.InfiniteLoveAndGratitude.com

"Health is a state of complete harmony of the body, mind and spirit. When one is free from physical disabilities and mental distractions, the gates of the soul open."
　　　　　　　　~ B.K.S. Iyengar

Simple Tips for Eating Healthy

Dori Babcock

There is so much information in the media today about eating right and nutrition—it's hard to make heads or tails of it all. We want to take care of ourselves—and it would be nice if it wasn't too much extra work. How do we know what is wrong and what is right? We hear that we should be eating this or drinking that, but how do we fit it in? How can our knowledge about healthy eating become our regular routine?

As an Exercise Physiologist and Wellness Coach, I am often asked for nutritional advice. Here are the questions I'm asked most frequently about nutrition. The answers offer five simple ways to a more nutritious lifestyle.

How can I eat more fruits and vegetables?
1. **Plan ahead.** Create a menu of fruits and vegetables you will eat for the day or week and stick to it.
2. **Have at least 3 colors of the rainbow in every meal.** Include fruits and/or vegetables in every meal. For example, make a low-fat yogurt smoothie for breakfast and throw in ½ cup of berries, peaches or bananas.
3. **Buy ready-to-eat** snacking vegetables like baby carrots and celery in the deli section of your local grocery store. Bag them up and put them in the fridge so they are ready to eat when you are.
4. **Add ½ - 1 cup of vegetables** or leafy greens to your pasta or rice dishes.
5. **Soups on!** Eat vegetable soup or soup with vegetables in it. Have you ever tried fruit soup? It's delicious—give it a try!

How can I prepare healthy meals fast?
1. **Stock your pantry,** your fridge, the breadbox and your freezer with spices and pantry standards such as pasta and rice that you can cook quickly. In your fridge always try to have two vegetables such as celery, carrots, peppers,

onions, broccoli, or lettuce available and don't forget condiments (salsa, pestos, mustards etc.). Dairy items can make a meal, such as cheese (cheddar, feta etc), yogurt, and skim milk. The breadbox could contribute whole wheat, French, and pita bread. In the freezer keep frozen vegetables, fruit juices, lean cuts of meat, Boboli pizza crust, and leftovers!

2. **Plan a menu.** What are your favorite meals? What ingredients do they have in common? If you prepare meals that have the same base vegetables, you can eat healthier and faster. For example, if you are cutting carrots for stir-fry on Monday, cut enough so that you can include them in pot roast for Tuesday and curry for Wednesday.

3. **Use your Crock Pot.** These truly are wonderful cooking tools. It is so nice to come home and smell the delicious dinner already made. All you need to add is a loaf of bread and a bag of green salad to complete the meal.

4. **Keep it simple.** Use a base of pasta, brown rice or other grain, toss in a cooked protein like grilled chicken or tofu, a few vegetables like steamed broccoli and carrots, then toss with low-fat dressing or sauce like teriyaki.

5. **Look for recipes.** Ask your friends if they have favorites to share. Go online and see what you can find that you will like.

How can I select a healthy option when eating out?

1. **Select lean cuts of red meat.** Sirloins and tenderloins are good choices; remove all visible traces of fat. For chicken and turkey, remove the skin before eating or ask for skinless portions.

2. **Look for the words** baked, broiled, steamed, poached, and roasted on the menu. Avoid meals that are sautéed, breaded, au gratin, fried or scalloped.

3. **Special order.** If there is not a healthy choice, ask if you can special order your entrée.

4. **On the Side.** Order any sauces or dressing on the side and dip your fork into them before taking a bite rather than pouring it over your dish or salad.

5. **Watch those portions!** A serving of meat is about the size of a deck of cards and a serving of pasta is about the size of your fist. Have your server box up half of your meal before bringing it to the table. You won't overeat and you'll have lunch the next day.

I'm trying to lose weight, what tips do you have for me?

1. **Drink water throughout the day.** It is easier for the body to shed fat when properly hydrated. You will also feel and have more energy and a better functioning digestive tract.

2. **Increase your vegetable, fruit, and fiber intake.** For example, eat more leafy greens and raw and steamed vegetables. Include fruit such as apples and pears and seeds like flax in your morning cereal and salads.

3. **Have a plan for tough food situations** such as free food at an office party or when someone pressures you, "One little piece won't hurt." Many a weight management plan has gone under from the office party and candy dish. Some strategies to follow are having some "treats" in your drawer, such as licorice that will satisfy your sweet tooth with lower calories. Take a different route around the candy dish. When someone presses you, tell them firmly, "No thank you" or, "I'll get some in a little while," and keep busy talking with someone else.

4. **Do not follow any recommendation that tells you** not to eat from an entire food group. Every food has a place in a well-balanced diet. Food is a pleasurable experience as well as fuel for our bodies. For example, simple carbohydrates are not very nutritious. These are white breads, pastas and rice. There is no need to remove these from the diet, just eat less of them. Instead of having 2 pieces of French bread and a second serving of spaghetti and pasta, choose one piece of bread and seconds on the salad with low-fat Italian dressing.

Simple Tips for Eating Healthy

5. **Eat five to six small meals throughout the day.** This will keep your blood sugar even, help stave off hunger, and allow you to try more fruits and vegetables as part of your regular diet.

Eating healthy does not have to be hard. The key to achievement is to start simple. Choose one or two of the simple changes above; work at making them a regular part of your lifestyle, and keep on going. Soon you will feel the benefits and reap the rewards of a healthy, balanced diet!

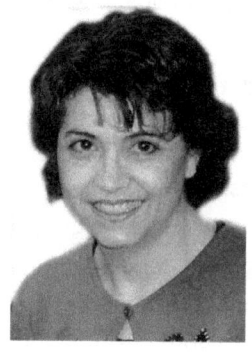

Dori Babcock is the director of the Northwest Health and Wellness Institute and formerly the Health and Wellness Consultant for the Weyerhaeuser Company's Excel Wellness Program. Dori has worked in health promotion for over 10 years and has a diverse background in patient-care, health education, health administration, conflict resolution, and worksite wellness. She has conducted research on access to preventive health services and has been published by the American Journal of Health Promotion. www.nhwinet.org

Getting Active? Start SMART!

Tara Zachgo

What do you think of when you hear the word "exercise"? Do you envision someone sweating and working out for hours in the gym? Some people have a negative association with the word "exercise." This is why it is often referred to as physical activity. It is recommended that people get some form of physical activity most days of the week. So, what is does this mean? Physical activity is any kind of movement which increases your heart rate. Examples would be aerobics class, manually mowing the lawn, gardening, walking, and even bowling. Now that we know the recommendation is to get our hearts pumping at a moderate intensity (breathing heavy but still able to talk) most days of the week, where do I start?

Getting started:

Step 1: Make a plan. A long-term plan can work, but only if you have developed one that is user-friendly and realistic. People want it all and want it now! This leads to a feeling of failure and giving up.

Step 2: Set goals, both short-term and long-term. Make sure your goals are SMART—specific, measurable, realistic, and timely. Focus on positive. For example, instead of "I am going to lose 20 pounds," change it to "I am going to walk for 15 minutes three times per week," and then increase the amount of time and/or days as you improve.

Step 3: Keep a journal or log. I know when I hold myself accountable by recording what I have done I am more successful. It gives you something to refer to where you can see your progress when you get frustrated or down on yourself. Look at what you have done so far.

Getting Active? Start SMART

Step 4: Reward your accomplishments. When establishing goals or target dates, have a reward in mind to strive towards. Reward yourself with small gifts along the way to keep you motivated.

Step 5: **Enjoy your active time!**

How to be successful when being active

The key is how you approach being active. If you think of it as another thing on your "to do" list it takes on a negative image like a chore. What kind of active personality do you have? The following are some questions to ask yourself when starting to implement an active lifestyle:

- Do I enjoy being alone or in a group setting?
- Do I enjoy the indoors or outdoors?
- Would I rather be active at home or away from home? If you choose home, are you able to focus on your active time or will you be distracted by the dirty dishes, laundry, bills, etc.? If you will be easily distracted you are setting yourself up to fail and make excuses, so away from home would be a better option.
- Do I like competition?
- Do I like to be adventurous?
- Do I like repetitiveness or change?
- Does activity energize me at the start of the day or relax me at the end of the day?

Think about these questions when you review your goals and choices of activities. The more you set your activities to your personal style, the more likely you are to stick to a plan and succeed.

Overcoming those barriers

We all have excuses as to why we are not more active. The key is to have a plan to counteract the excuse from the start. The most common complaint is "I don't have time to be active." Well, there are 1440 minutes in a day—most people can spare at least 30 minutes to be active. You do not have to be active for 30 continuous minutes. Break it up into smaller segments if that is all your schedule allows. Walk over the lunch hour, during meetings, walk to co-workers instead of e-mailing, use the stairs, etc. Some people have all the right intentions of getting active and then something "better" comes along so they skip out on their active time. Mark your time in your calendar. Make it an appointment. Plan ahead. You write down meeting times and doctor's appointments. You would have a negative consequence if you missed these scheduled times; treat your active time the same way. Don't punish yourself because you missed one day. Just start up again the next day or scheduled time. It will take about 6 weeks for you to adapt to a schedule and have it become part of your daily routine. At about 6 months your active lifestyle will become a healthy habit. The time to be healthy is now!

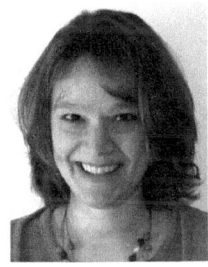

Tara L. Zachgo graduated with a Bachelor of Science Degree in Kinesiology from Kansas State University. She is a Certified Medical Assistant, a Certified/Licensed Athletic Trainer, and a Certified Lifestyle Fitness Coach. She currently works as a Health Promotion Clinical Specialist at Fort HealthCare located in Fort Atkinson, Wisconsin. She is applying her experience as the Corporate Wellness Coordinator of Fort HealthCare to Community Wellness Initiatives in the Fort HealthCare service area. www.forthealthcare.com

"I see rejection in my skin, worry in my cancers, bitterness and hate in my aching joints. I failed to take care of my mind, and so my body now goes to hospital."
~ Astrid Alauda

Are We Sitting Comfortably? Then Let's Begin

Leslie Kahn

We seek comfort in many forms: from comfortable clothes and blankets to feelings of peace and restfulness. Why should we not have comfort in our everyday work environment? The American Heritage Dictionary defines comfortable as "Providing physical comfort; free from stress or anxiety; at ease; producing feelings of ease or security." [1]

Is it possible to have comfort in the place where I work? Some of us spend a majority of our day in a sitting position, moving from one desk or meeting table to another. In one week, those hours can add up fast to a total of 12 to 30 hours.

In a seated position, we sometimes become sore and fatigued. Those headaches, back pain, sore arms and fingers could be caused by how we approach our desk and workstations. If you're like me, you just plop down in the chair and adjust the height, never giving any thought to your desk height, arm rest, monitor, or how your body is positioned. When I had muscle pain or fatigue, I used to think, "Am I getting old or sick?" I really needed to start with my environment—which was my chair, desk, and monitor and look at how I was positioning myself.

Here's how we can sit comfortably at work. Let's begin by talking about the neutral position. The neutral position is a working position where your joints are naturally aligned. This reduces stress and strain on the muscles, tendons, and skeletal system and reduces your risk of musculoskeletal injury such as carpal tunnel syndrome and tendonitis.

Right now, take a look at the way your workstation is set up:

---

[1] comfortable. (n.d.). The American Heritage® Dictionary of the English Language, Fourth Edition. Retrieved October 09, 2008, from Dictionary.com website: http://dictionary.reference.com/browse/comfortable

Are We Sitting Comfortably? Then Let's Begin

- Is your computer monitor at eye level so that your head and neck are in a neutral position (not looking down or up)?
- Do you have a good, comfortable, adjustable chair? Do you even know how to adjust your good, comfortable chair?
- Is your telephone positioned so that you do not have to twist your back when you answer it?
- Is your mouse in a position that allows your wrist to be in a neutral position?
- Do you have a slanted document holder so that you are not reading off of a flat surface when transposing material to your computer?
- Is your desk at the right height for you?

Consider these while trying to maintain neutral body positions at your computer workstation:

1. Hands, wrists, and forearms are straight, in-line and parallel to the floor
2. The head is level or bent slightly forward, facing forward and balanced; the head is aligned above the torso and neck. Avoid sticking your head and neck out toward the monitor
3. The shoulders are relaxed and before you begin working, the upper arms hang comfortably at your side
4. The elbows stay close in toward the body and are bent between 90 and 120 degrees
5. The feet are flat on the floor, fully supported; a footrest should be used if the desk height is not adjustable
6. The back is fully supported, using a lumbar support if necessary, and you are sitting vertically
7. The thighs and hips are supported by a well-padded seat, parallel to the floor; Make sure there is ample room between the end of the seat and the backs of the knees.
8. The knees are the same height as the hips.

With these few changes to our workstation, we can begin to alleviate the effects of bad posture. Here are some bonus tips to increase their effectiveness. This will help to enhance the results of what we're already doing right to sit comfortably.

Move Around During the Day

It's easy to become engrossed in what you are working on at your computer and then realize that you have been sitting in one place for three hours. I do it myself sometimes. The human body was not designed to sit for long periods; certainly not for 14 hours a day. Just think about how your back feels when you do get up. Now, remember that feeling. To avoid a very stiff back and legs, make sure you stand up AT LEAST every hour. A five-minute break every half hour would be better and a one-minute break every 10–15 minutes would be even better.

Vary Your Tasks

Vary your tasks throughout the day. When you take a break from your computer, take a walk and use the copier. Make some telephone calls, but not when you are sitting at your computer. It is highly recommended that you stand up for part of the day rather than sitting all day; there are height adjustable workstations.

STRETCH!

Stretching throughout the day will reduce muscle tension, improve circulation, reduce anxiety, stress and fatigue, improve mental alertness, decrease the risk of injury, and make you feel good. There is software that reminds you when, how, and what to stretch. There are several websites that demonstrate office stretches. No excuses anymore.

Avoid Eye Strain

Your eyes get tired, too, staring at the computer screen for long periods. Make sure you periodically look out the window or look at a distant object. This allows your eyes to rest from constant close-up work.

Telephone Neck

In this 21st century of multi-tasking, many of us talk on the telephone while we are typing at our computers. This leads to the dreaded cradling of the telephone between the ear and the shoulder. Ouch! GET A HEADSET if you spend a lot of time on the telephone. Better yet, get a wireless headset so that you can stand up and move around while you are talking. Think of all the oxygen getting to your brain. You'll think more clearly.

By making the effort to design your work environment for maximum productivity, you can avoid fatigue and discomfort. Our time at work should energize us to some degree and allow for more positive interactions with our co-workers, customers and clients.

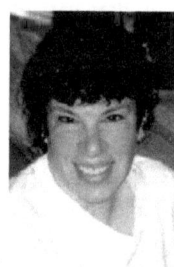

Leslie Kahn, a member of the American Massage Therapy Association, is a state licensed massage therapist and a graduate of the Chicago School of Massage Therapy, August 1996. Leslie and her husband, Martin Aistrope, the Humor Therapist member of KneadaLaugh, have an 8-year-old adopted son who supplies them with all their best material.   www.kneadalaugh.com

Section 2: Intellectual Wellness

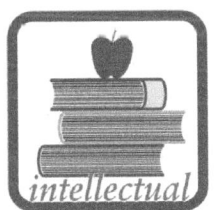

"The world is endless, the universe inexhaustible, and the human brain will never be threatened with unemployment."
*~ Genrich Altshuller,
    The Innovation Algorithm*

Section 2: Intellectual Wellness

Introduction

Intellectual Wellness is the desire to learn from challenges and past experiences. It seeks methods for intellectual growth and creative mental activities that provide the foundation to discover, process, and evaluate information. Intellectual wellness can be achieved by finding resources to expand our knowledge and improve our decision-making skills.

Characteristics of Intellectual Wellness:

- Concentration and focus
- Problem solving techniques
- Creativity
- Goals for education and learning in personal and professional areas
- Critical thinking capability
- Ability to adapt to change and access necessary resources

Continually learning from the best resources available stimulates our minds and enables us to become more capable of analyzing the world around us. We must begin to stretch ourselves to increase our companionship with noteworthy people, books, cultures, and works of art. Only then can we begin to take advantage of the great opportunities that lie ahead of us.

The Need for Intellectual Wellness

Did you know that ...

"According to a 2003 study by the National Association of Manufacturers (NAM): 'The Skills Gap: Manufacturers Confront Persistent Skills Shortages in an Uncertain Economy,' more than 80% of manufacturers reported a "moderate to serious" shortage of qualified applicants; even though more than two million manufacturing layoffs occurred during the recent recession.

Intellectual Wellness

"And it's just going to get worse. The study also reports that by the year 2020, the deficit of skilled workers in the United States will reach 10 million. Companies need to recruit and train new workers now, so they can become technically proficient and gain some of the older, more experienced workers' knowledge before the baby boomers' mass exodus from the workforce begins."

Training & Education Mastery: Alltech, Debra Kelly,
Copyright © 2007 Thomas Publishing Company

Bill Gates had this to say about the state of education in America:

"When I compare our high schools to what I see when I'm traveling abroad, I am terrified for our work force of tomorrow," he said.

"Only one-third of our students graduate from high school ready for college, work and citizenship," he said. Gates spoke bluntly about the high dropout rates in America compared with those of other developed countries, and the differences between America's high-tech graduate degrees and those in India and China."

Gates "appalled" by high schools,
The Seattle Times, February 27, 2005

"Managers (and all employees) must take responsibility for their own learning. At one time, many companies could promise a new employee lifelong employment and a predictable career path. Today, very few if any companies can make that promise. Even when your company has a formal training department and offers a catalog full of courses for employees, no one knows better than the employee and his or her manager what needs to be learned and how that learning can be applied to the job to make a positive difference in individual, group, and company business results. You must take responsibility for your own career path, whether with your current employer or through a series of employers. And the way to build your career is to keep learning throughout your career."

Take Responsibility for Your Own Learning,
Copyright ©1998 Daniel R. Tobin

Intellectual Wellness Experts

In this section, your wellness vision turns into reality with the help of Merrilee Shopland, "Your Wellness Vision: Turning Resolutions into Reality." Step through a plan with Merrilee and be successful in reaching and sticking to your goal.

Then, Anne Ward and Bob Sandidge tell us how to use our brain's natural abilities to increase our focus in "The Energizing Power of Focus." They also recommend that we sprint through our busy days.

Next, Dr. Andrea Brockman discusses how eliminating Dental Stress leverages the effectiveness of Wellness Programs. Dr. Brockman raises our dental I.Q. to improve our overall health and wellness. Learn why dental ignorance is not bliss.

Finally, we understand the importance of wellness coaching with Billie Jo Hance and Diana Stratigakis. Wellness coaches become our partners for health improvement and accountability. They help us leverage our current strengths and set us on a healthful journey of improvement.

Let's begin!

Intellectual Wellness: Personal Assessment

Read the questions and rate yourself from 0 (low level) to 5 (high level) of achievement. Determine the total number for each rating and compare it to the answer key below. This determines where your intellectual wellness stands today. Take the test again in 30 days to check your progress on improving intellectual wellness. Remember, improvement in any area is *positive action in motion*.

1. I have a professional coach who leads me through dips in my development.

    5   4   3   2   1   0

Intellectual Wellness

2. I am a continual learner of information via magazines, books, Internet, or seminars.

    5   4   3   2   1   0

3. I am able to focus on the task at hand with limited distractions.

    5   4   3   2   1   0

4. I'm open-minded and willing to see things from a different point of view.

    5   4   3   2   1   0

5. I learn from my challenges and experiences.

    5   4   3   2   1   0

6. I look for ways to innovate and create opportunities for my organization.

    5   4   3   2   1   0

7. I seek opportunities to combine work with community so both benefit.

    5   4   3   2   1   0

8. I am regarded as someone others want on their teams.

    5   4   3   2   1   0

9. I am the "go to" person for work related challenges or opportunities.

    5   4   3   2   1   0

10. I search for ways to personally grow.

    5   4   3   2   1   0

Answer Key: If you answered,

Mostly 5's you have an excellent level of intellectual wellness. Continue stretching your comfort zone and finding ways to gain greater benefits of being intellectually fit. Consider teaching others how they can reach their intellectual wellness goals.

Mostly 4's you have a high level of intellectual wellness. Consider finding innovative ways to make your 4's turn to 5's. This can be fun and exciting.

Mostly 3's you have a reasonable level of intellectual wellness. With a greater attempt and laser focus, you become the model of what it takes to get where you want to be.

Mostly 2's you're at a good starting point of intellectual wellness. Allow yourself to begin again, set goals and go for it!

Mostly 1's it's time for an upgrade. You have what it takes. Make yourself a priority. Wellness is important to thrive and survive in todays fast pace world.

Mostly 0's choose one area of intellectual wellness to improve upon each month. Seek a buddy to help you find ways to reach your goal, hold you accountable and be your cheerleader. You're worth the investment!

"The I in illness is isolation, and the crucial letters in wellness are we."

~ Author unknown, as quoted in Mimi Guarneri, The Heart Speaks: A Cardiologist Reveals the Secret Language of Healing

Your Wellness Vision: Turning Resolutions into Reality

Merrilee Shopland, M.A.

Never get on a scale during a vacation. I did that one Spring Break and afterwards every roll, pat of butter, and glance at the dessert tray was a trip down Guilt Avenue. But the antidote to guilt is action and I vowed right away to do something about it later, after the vacation. Now I am well familiar with the recipe for health behavior change. I teach kinesiology at a college and each semester I guide the students towards accomplishing one health goal. I teach six steps to making a health resolution a reality. But teaching it is not the same as doing it. Could I walk the talk?

First step: Start with the end in mind. You may think I stole this one from Stephen Covey, but I actually learned it from an Entertainment Producer who said you always start planning from the day something is finished and work backwards. So I set about creating my S.M.A.R.T. goal: one that is Specific, Measurable, Accessible, Relevant and Time-Sensitive. Now here's an important tip: It needs to be visual. I knew I needed to lose about 15 pounds and at least 2 inches off of my hips and I wanted that to happen by August 1st—but what really helped was my VISION. I saw myself running out of the ocean with a black two-piece swimsuit on (wasn't even thinking bikini) and yelling to my husband and son, "Come on in, the water is great!" and running back "Bay Watch" style into the blue-green waters of the Caribbean.

Which brings me to the **second step: Picture a Payoff.** When you hit the obstacles, the inner whining, the detours, the saboteurs with their happy hours and chocolate cake in the break room, you need to have an image of a payoff that will get you to home plate. This needs to be something you would not ordinarily give yourself. Something pivotally marvelous.

Now we come to the step people want to skip: the **third step: Assess Your Current Situation.** Think about the behaviors that sabotage your good intentions in regards to your health goal. Then write down the costs and benefits associated with that behavior. For example, if you like your evening wine, analyze both rewards . . . relaxation, fun . . . as well as the downside to the behavior, such as your discipline slipping, added calories, temptation to go out to eat. Do the benefits outweigh the costs? Is there something you could do that would achieve the same benefit? Perhaps the benefits are too great during this stressful period of your life. Maybe now is not the time to make the change. Or you could find out what I found out when I did the exercise, that the costs were tearing apart the fabric of my self-esteem.

It's helpful to understand your true readiness to make this change and you might want to Google Prochaska's and DiClemente's Stages of Change Model. These two psychologists theorized that behavior change is not an event but a process that unfolds over months and years and is characterized by five distinct stages: Pre-contemplation, Contemplation, Preparation, Action and Maintenance. This model views an unsuccessful attempt to change not as failure but as an opportunity to learn how to sustain change more effectively in the future. Are you really ready to change is an important thing to know.

Because I teach exercise—in front of a group of young college students who, weirdly enough, seem frozen in that 18–21 year-old timeline, while I'm rushing headlong into my fifties—I'm motivated to change. Ok, here it comes, the critical one, **step number four: Create a Strong Strategy.** I call it WWW. What will you be doing to affect this change; Where will you be doing it, and When? It has to be on the schedule. So here's what it looked like for me: I jump up my exercise regimen at the gym from four to five times a week. I go to and join Weight Watchers. Now I am not a Weight Watcher's type. I don't like the idea, the format, or the group clapping. But I armor myself with a friend and we sit in the back row and laugh a lot. I count points, nachos, and the pounds that are dropping off. I tell my husband NOT to ask me to get pizza or Mexican food. I inform my Mom before I go over that she is not to ask me if I want dessert. I buy a great exercise outfit—with plenty of spandex. I buy an mp3 player to exercise to and a journal for writing about my process. I write a note on the fridge: "What you need is not in here." What I'm talking about is lining up your support. You're going to need some allies for this endeavor.

So far you have your goal, your payoff, you've analyzed your current situation, and you find you are ready to change. So you line up your support, and you devise a strategy that would impress General Patton. What's left? Oh yeah, the obstacles. Didn't Obi-Wan Kenobi warn you? There's always a big, bad something around the corner that's going to ask you if you want this bad enough. There's even a voice inside of us that tells us it's too darn hard. Is your payoff big enough to traverse the rugged terrain? This is when you get out those benefits and plaster them somewhere you can see them every day. **Step number five: Anticipate the Obstacles.**

Step number six is waking up every day and remembering what you are going for, why you are doing it, what strategy and support will help you, and dealing with the challenges that arise in your journey towards health. In other words, **step number six is Working the Plan you have created** and focusing on the purpose of this health challenge you have taken on. "Happiness can be defined, in part at least, as the fruit of the desire to sacrifice what we want now for what we want eventually." Now I did steal that one from Stephen Covey.

That year I went on another vacation, 18 pounds lighter, and I found myself in the ocean marveling at the beauty and power of the waves. As each wave came, I would jump up into the air, into the sunlight, having a blast in my new black, velvet, two-piece swimsuit. My husband and son sat on the beach for longer than I expected. Impatient and excited, I ran on to the shore up to my family gushing about how great the water was and to hurry up and come in. They looked appalled. As I turned around to go back in, I discovered my top had slid way too far off the target. Oops. So life isn't perfect. And it wasn't the Caribbean. It was New Jersey. But the vision that had miraculously and somewhat imperfectly manifested had gotten me to my goal.

Changing our health is not necessarily easy. The cost of discipline, clarity, and courage can be steep. But this isn't just about our health, it is about our relationship to ourselves, about creating a life that is vital and authentic to who we feel we really are. My small battle with 18 pounds still remains one of my favorite victories, and the picture of the payoff manifesting brings a definite smile.

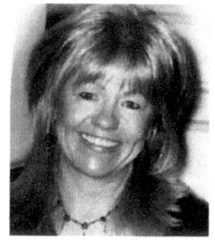**Merrilee Shopland**, M.A. has been an educator and speaker in the wellness industry since 1985. She ran a holistic fitness center for women over 30 and an eight-campus college wellness program in Austin, Texas. Merrilee has taught Kinesiology in Higher Education for the past 18 years and is certified by the American Council on Exercise. Her background also includes work in multimedia and theatrical presentation, where she has written and produced online tutorials, musicals and films. merrilee@austincc.edu
www.austincc.edu/shopland

The Energizing Power of Focus

Anne Ward and Bob Sandidge

I'd like you to do a quick experiment while you're reading the rest of this paragraph: just tap your finger or your foot while reading. No particular rhythm, just let your hand or foot tap out whatever it does. I'll make a prediction about how this works out for you: I'll bet you're a star at multitasking when one of your tasks is purely cognitive (reading the words on the page) and one is purely physical (allowing your finger or foot to tap to its own beat). You didn't miss a single word once you got the tapping going, did you?

Now, try this experiment: as you're reading this paragraph, tap out the beat of the song "Happy Birthday" while singing the words silently in your head. Start now. There has been quite a bit of research in the last 10 years about the brain's ability to multitask when it comes to paying attention. The brain can only focus on one concept at a time. When you try to pay attention to more than one concept, project, person, or line of thought at the same time, your brain looks at each sequentially, not simultaneously.[1] OK, you can stop singing now. So how did your experiment go? Did you need to read any of the sentences more than once while you were singing in your head? Did you need to stop singing in order to get the full meaning of the words you were reading?

So, can human beings multitask? Based on the results of these experiments, yes...and no. When only one of the tasks involves active, conscious attention, you're likely to be able to accomplish both tasks without either one suffering too much. Other examples of multitasking where only one of the tasks involves conscious attention:

- Eating lunch while reading a book
- Preparing a simple recipe you've made many times while talking to a friend

---

[1] Rubinstein, J. S., Meyer, D. E., & Evans, J. E. (2001). Executive control of cognitive processes in task switching. *Journal of Experimental Psychology: Human Perception and Performance, 27,* 763-797

- Walking a dog while taking on a cell phone

The difficulty with multitasking comes when we try to do two things at one time, both of which require conscious cognitive processing. For example:

- Thinking about what you're supposed to do next while listening to and remembering someone's name
- Attempting a complicated new recipe while trying to hold a conversation
- Writing a report while thinking about tomorrow's meeting

In each of these situations, we know from studies that our brains will go back and forth between the two tasks (so imagine if you add in a ringing phone, your boss calling you, and the emotional pull from last night's romantic dinner with an exciting new person in your life). Humans are not biologically capable of paying active, conscious attention to two concepts at once. When we attempt to do so, we now know that we will process our tasks 50% more slowly and that we will make up to 50% more errors.[2]

When you can truly focus on the one important thing in front of you, are vastly more productive and your work is of higher quality with fewer errors. Multitasking steals your ability to focus.

In today's world, what can you do to increase focus?

Since multitasking doesn't work, yet we live in a world where it seems to be valued—indeed required—how can we protect our ability to produce an abundance of quality work results? I've put together this list, also based on research about how our brains work, that will give you some ideas about how to add more focus to your work and your life.

---

[2] Medina, John, Brain Rules, Pear Press, 2008, p 87

Automatic Cognitive Thieves

Watch out for these types of thoughts that can worm their way into your mind and steal your focus away:

Worry. It's insidious, takes your mind off of what you're doing, and pretends to be important. It demands acknowledgment and usually gets it because we tend to worry about things that affect us emotionally which trigger an automatic attention response. But worry itself does nothing for us. If you realize that something needs to be done, make a note and schedule the act. If there's nothing you can do, acknowledge the emotion behind the worry and either return your attention to what you're working on or (in tough cases) schedule time to do some really good worrying later.

Thinking about the Past or the Future. "If things had only been different..." "If everything goes right next week..." Imagine you're in a beautiful landscape looking through a pair of binoculars. You adjust the lenses so you can clearly see the mountain in the far distance as if it was just a few steps away. When you move the binoculars a bit, notice that the trees in front of the mountain are now so out of focus you can only make out a hazy green blur. You simply can't keep both what's in front of you and what's far away—far in front of you or far behind—in focus at the same time either with your binoculars or with your mind. While it's good to check in with the past in order to learn and with the future in order to set your course, it's the step you make now that will actually take you where you're going. When the past or future entices you on an unplanned journey, refocus on what's right in front of you. Life can only be lived now.

Should. Whenever you hear this word in your head, sound an alarm. You are being pulled into another dimension from which escape can be difficult. Once you get going, it's easy to get caught up in a hundred tributaries that go nowhere. No doubt the world is unfair, things happen that no one would prefer, and, well, it just isn't right. Now...what were you working on that will actually move you toward your next goal?

The Energizing Power of Focus

To reduce your Automatic Cognitive Thieves, you need to become aware of them first. I recommend tracking them for a week or so. Just put a mark on a piece of paper every time you notice one and then return to what you were doing.

Sprinting vs. Running a Marathon

Sprinters and marathoners both run, but the sports themselves are quite different. Sprinters run full-out for a short distance in a short period of time. Marathoners pace themselves to conserve energy for the long road ahead. Sprinting requires strength and, because sprinting has both aerobic and anaerobic components, sprinting actually builds strength and capacity. Running a marathon requires endurance—the ability to keep going long after one feels he simply can't go any farther. Both skills are valuable. While there will be times in your life where you'll be required to go an incredible distance and your endurance will be tested, most of what life asks of you will be better met by learning to sprint.

Research that started with sleep studies shows that our brains (and bodies) function in natural cycles through the day and night—what are known as ultradian rhythms. Each cycle is about 90–120 minutes long and builds to a peak of activity and awareness, then drops again before the next cycle.[3] Sport psychologists help athletes train more effectively and more efficiently by teaching them to take advantage of these natural cycles. And now business people are learning to plan their work as a series of sprints through the workday with periods of rest in between. According to Jim Loehr, "...The richer and deeper the source of emotional recovery, the more we refill our reserves and the more resilient we become. Effective emotional renewal puts us in a position to perform more effectively, especially under pressure."[4] The rest periods between work "sprints" can include things that recharge your mental and physical batteries: grabbing a healthy snack, going for a walk, having an engaging conversation, reading something interesting, energizing

---

[3] Rossi, Ernest Lawrence Ph.D., The 20 Minute Break, Jeremy P. Tarcher, 1991 p 17

[4] Loehr, Jim and Schwartz, Tony, The Power of Full Engagement, The Free Press, 2003, p 77

or inspirational. Things that would not be recommended are reading email, surfing the Internet, watching TV, eating high sugar or high sodium snacks, or going over your to-do list.

Try to fit two or more 90-minute sprints into your day followed by re-energizing breaks and see if you get more high quality work done.

Keep Your Head in the Game

We do live in a world of interruptions and competing priorities, so what else can a person do when the demand for multitasking seems overwhelming?

Get it Out of Your Head. You need a good capture tool, a place where you can make a note of what you need to remember without taking a lot of time out of your current focus priority. Some people use notepads (use only one notepad for all capture, not multiple notes in different places), others use digital recorders or day planners.

Know Your Short List. Write down the three to five goals that are most important to you right now. You may think of them as tasks or projects, but for the Short List, write them as if they were already accomplished. This allows your subconscious mind to work on them even when you're consciously doing something else.

Watch for Goal Creep. Once you have your Short List, code every item on your daily task list by which important goal it relates to directly or indirectly. If an item on the list is not related to your Short List, to what goal is it related? Do this for a couple of weeks. It will help you see when you're in danger of over-committing to more goals than you can handle in high quality fashion.

Scrutinize Randomness. When unplanned items come up through the day, write them down and relate them to your goals before you actually do them. Do this for a few days from time to time. It's a good check-in with your priorities that will help to keep you on track.

Your ability to focus on what's important to you will give you a life of meaningful accomplishment. So watch out for people who want you to tap your foot while singing songs.

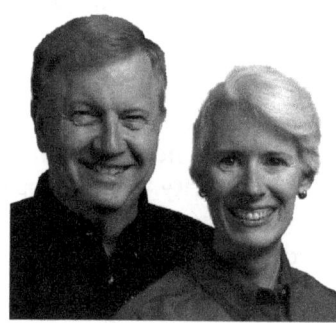

Anne Ward and Bob Sandidge are change agents, authors, trainers, facilitators, holistic marketers and creative consultants who have worked in the realms of Change, Growth, Communications, Holistic Marketing, and Organizational and Personal Transformation since 1991. Anne is currently working on a book about FOCUS of attention. Both are NLP Trainers and Practitioners.

CreativeCore.com   NLPeople.com

Eliminating Dental Stress Leverages Wellness

Andrea H. Brockman, RN, DDS

Do you remember how excited you were when you lost your first tooth and how gratifying it was when the last one came out? Teething was uncomfortable, but it was a rite of passage. Our teeth surely opened our world to food, communication, sex appeal, and protection. It's curious that earlier in life, we celebrate teeth coming in and falling out, but as adults we often underestimate their true value. We take care of our gums and teeth because it makes us feel and look good. And we enjoy eating. But let's face it; even though the oral cavity represents the first stage of the digestive process - which from a medical standpoint can and does have a significant bearing on the later stages of digestion - physicians rarely address dental conditions mostly because their medical training just doesn't include it. And since medical insurance doesn't cover dental work, (even for health reasons), gums, teeth, and jaws, when compared with other organs and systems in the body, appear not to be so important for health and longevity. Nothing is further from the truth. Oral health and stability are essential to wellness.

The Mouth is Not an Independent Entity

What's so remarkable, having been an intensive care nurse before I went to dental school, is witnessing the absolute lack of interest and attention among nurses and physicians when it comes to dentistry. It's almost as if the mouth were not a part of the rest of the body. But I couldn't forget my nursing training and ministering to the whole person when I treated my dental patients. People always asked me why I didn't become a physician. My reasons were practical. I wanted to stay in healthcare but decided that I needed a change from the intensive care and later geriatric work environment to work with relatively healthy people. Ironically, my hospital experiences uniquely prepared me to treat the dental needs of critically or chronically ill people. So those who had heart attacks, organ transplants, cancer, MS, diabetes, and every other ailment ended up being my dental patients.

For over 25 years I looked at my dental patients' medical histories and often observed oral symptoms from their systemic problems. And not so surprising to me, many seemed to show improvement in emotional and physical health and well-being with dental interventions. In my practice, referrals back and forth to physicians were commonplace. The doctors thought that there were less post-op infections and pneumonia when patients got their teeth and gums cleaned before surgery. Many chronic sinus problems dissipated when we diagnosed and treated infected upper teeth. I repeatedly saw patients burdened by debilitating headaches, back, and neck pain get relief from dental treatment. And women needing dental work during their pregnancy who recognized the consequences of tobacco, alcohol, and caffeine, also chose dental restorative materials that would not be potentially harmful to their fetus.

Ignorance is not Bliss

While more and more studies on the links of periodontal disease to heart attacks, strokes, diabetes, pre-term births, and low-birth weight babies are surfacing every day, I'm still amazed that manufacturers of oral care products don't stress this in their advertising. Commercials and magazine articles emphasize plaque reduction for fresher breath. Desirable yes, but germs in the mouth do a lot more damage than cause bad breath. The doctors, the heart association, and the dental association could be doing more to engage the public and the medical community. Pity the uninformed people with untreated periodontal disease whose ignorance could sentence them to early death.

It's not enough to tell people they need to see their dentist more regularly or even provide a dental insurance benefit. For years, dentists have been less than 50% successful using a number of strategies and incentives to keep patients regularly returning for maintenance visits. People may postpone or forego treatment if dental expenditures exceed allowable insurance. The statistics from dental insurance claims show that even with 100% coverage for preventive services, utilization is appallingly low. Going to the dentist may be one of life's least pleasant experiences, but paying for dentistry can be downright excruciating.

The Costs of Health

From both a health and economic perspective, employers must consider that when the body is healthy, the gums and teeth also do well. Compliance in wellness programs may very well increase if people, who want to lose weight, decrease their stress, and stop smoking would also learn about oral-systemic health connections that could save them from needing costly and uncomfortable dental treatment. That may prove to be a much greater incentive than a gift card or free lunch.

It's no secret that enormous rate hikes in health insurance premiums resulted from increased medical utilization. Employers now recognize that it makes incredibly more economic sense to avoid health problems than it does to treat them. Therefore, wellness and disease management programs are absolutely essential for the health of their business. And dentistry leverages each one of those programs for higher yield.

Dental Stressors to Health

In order to understand this concept, I have created a model called The Health Stressor Index, which is the foundation of the HealthyGates Dental Risk Assessment, a self-questionnaire. Physical and emotional stressors can overwhelm us by their assault or cause deficiencies of things essential to support health. Examples of some stressors include trauma, lack of nutrients, lack of physical activity, infections, toxic exposures, structural imbalance, emotional stress, sleep disturbances, medications, drug and alcohol abuse, smoking, and dental stress. Each individual stressor varies in strength and duration and they add on to one another. Depending on the nature of one's constitution and genetic makeup, the threshold for coping with the buildup of stressors varies and is unknown. Some people have a greater capacity to adapt. One stressor is rarely the entire cause of illness and conversely, removing or lessening a stressor does not guarantee a cure. However, most agree that reducing any stressor is a positive health choice. Here we will consider the dental stressor and its impact on several health conditions.

Understand that a clean mouth is not the sole benchmark for dental health. Other dental conditions such as infections, jaw imbalances, and toxic dental materials can stress the health and well-being of the entire body. Since dentists can't practice medicine and physicians pretty much ignore dental conditions, there is a void in healthcare. Wellness coordinators who provide dental-systemic health education and assess dental stressors can play a very important role in vastly improving workplace health and the company's bottom line.

Raising Dental IQ Improves Overall Health

Many well thought out wellness programs are set up to reduce the risks for heart disease and diabetes. Health risk assessments and laboratory tests help to determine if blood pressure, cholesterol levels, body mass, smoking habits, and activity qualify an employee to enroll in any number of programs. While medications help keep laboratory indicators within acceptable limits, fitness, nutritional counseling, smoking cessation, and stress management require change, discipline, and long-term commitment. But ignored or unrecognized relentless dental distress can undermine the gains. Here are a few examples.

Obesity may have a bit to do with food selection. There could be a dental component such as missing teeth or painful gums or inadequate salivary flow that would make soft starchy foods easier to eat. Improper chewing of proteins could exacerbate digestive problems and prevent absorption of proper nutrients.

Heart attack risks increase with periodontal disease. Diabetics and smokers have a higher incidence of gum disease thereby further increasing their risk for a heart attack and stroke.

Sleep disturbances cause fatigue and affect decisions, mood, and safety in the workplace. Oral soft tissue structures may be involved.

Headaches, neck, and back pain can affect productivity and attendance. Common, but overlooked dental influences may be bite or jaw imbalance, clenching or grinding, tooth movement, and dental pain from teeth, gums, jawbone, or TMJ.

Allergies and chemical sensitivities may be aggravated by dental materials that may not be compatible with the immune system.

Pregnancy complications such as preterm birth and low birth weight babies are possibilities with untreated gum disease. Mercury vapor released from placing, drilling out, or polishing dental amalgam fillings can pass through placenta and breast milk.

Athletic performance such as flexibility, endurance, hand-eye coordination, and recovery from injury can be affected by dental infections, jaw imbalances, and toxic restorative materials.

Emotional stress may take its toll on the mouth manifesting in broken teeth, worn dentition, sensitive teeth, jaw pain, facial pain, mouth ulcers, and less resistance to oral infections.

Wellness coordinators can play a very important role in increasing employee awareness of health-related dental conditions by providing all workers with a comprehensive dental risk assessment. They should also incorporate oral-systemic health education into each wellness and disease management endeavor to help leverage the program for improved attendance and productivity. The addition of this health-promoting knowledge can ultimately reduce medical claims and advance wellness for the long term.

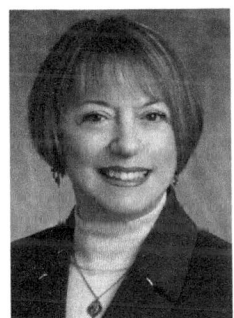

Dr. Andrea Brockman is President of OraMedica International, LLC a wellness company founded in 2003 devoted to helping improve total health through knowledge of the dental connections to chronic disease, pain, obesity, and stress. She is a 1979 graduate of Temple Dental School and has her undergraduate degree in Nursing from Temple University. Dr. Brockman is the author of employee dental health tips booklets, the HealthyGates dental risk assessment and series of dental information e-books. She consults with companies and provides executive training for incorporating oral-systemic education into wellness programs. www.oramedica.com

"If you have health, you probably will be happy, and if you have health and happiness, you have all the wealth you need, even if it is not all you want."
   ~ *Elbert Hubbard*

Wellness Coaching:
Partnering to Make Positive Changes

Diana Stratigakis and Billie Jo Hance

Today, companies are looking for ways to keep their employees healthier, happier, and ultimately, more engaged. Employees, on the other hand, often find that their companies don't connect meaningfully with them as they struggle to balance work and family while maintaining their health, managing their weight and stress, and finding time to exercise. Recently however, wellness coaching has become a popular method for bringing about positive changes in employee health and wellness. Unlike the "expert" model which, paradoxically, tends to make people feel less in control of their health and wellness, coaching identifies and builds on employee strengths.[1] A session with a coach can identify the areas an employee feels ready and motivated to change and create a supportive partnership to help the employee move toward his vision of wellness.

Employees who participate in wellness coaching are seeing meaningful results. Take Care Health Solutions, a subsidiary of Walgreens Corporation, designs and implements coaching and other wellness programs for a variety of organizations. In one client organization, results of a de-identified, aggregate cohort group of 5000 employees demonstrated how health coaching can help employees move out of high and very high risk groups into low and moderate risk. The program offers biometrics (weight, body fat and body mass index), a health assessment, a cholesterol and blood glucose screening, and coaching. According to a client representative, "Coaching sessions provide an optimal setting to talk about identified risk factors and support the formulation of goals. Coaches prepare the employee to address challenges that might be barriers for reaching those goals. Discussions between coaches and employees are motivational and focus on long-term behavior change." Employees often report that the most helpful aspect of

---

[1] Moore, M and Boothroyd, L. The Obesity Epidemic: A confidence crisis calling for professional coaches, Wellesley, MA: Wellcoaches Corporation, 2006.

their coaching experience is having someone to whom they can be accountable.

Wellness coaching is defined as "a close relationship and partnership with a coach providing the structure, accountability, expertise, and inspiration to enable an individual to learn, grow, and develop beyond what s/he can do alone." [2] Wellness coaches help clients lose weight, begin or maintain an exercise program, incorporate better eating habits, manage stress, improve their general health, and achieve a better work/life balance.

Employees are often unsure about what to expect from a coaching session. When it comes to their health, they are used to simply being told what to do by their doctor. Coaches may find their clients caught off guard—but often pleasantly surprised—when they are treated as a partner in the coaching process. In a coaching session, the client is considered to have expert knowledge of how best to reach his or her own goals. Therefore, the coach only acts as an expert when absolutely necessary, for example, when the client needs additional information in order to move forward.

The following examples illustrate this shift in thinking:

- Traditional: How long has it been since you exercised?
- Coach: What did it feel like when you were exercising regularly?
- Traditional: You should exercise to lower your blood pressure.
- Coach: What do you know about the connection between exercise and your blood pressure?
- Traditional: If you cut out soda and junk food, you will lose the 5 pounds a month you want to lose.
- Coach: What could you commit to doing this week that would help you move toward your vision of losing weight?

---

[2] Moore, M, ed., Wellcoaches Training Manual. Wellesley, MA: Wellcoaches Corporation; 2004.

Coaches come from a variety of backgrounds—counseling, fitness, dietetics, nursing, and health education—but are united by the approach they take to working with clients. The basis for this unified approach is that coaching is client driven. The coach's main goal is to work with the client's agenda, rather than to prescribe a solution to a problem. Through a process of active listening, asking questions, and reflecting back what is heard, coaches draw out from their clients how they would like to move forward. In this way, coaching is distinct from other behavior change strategies. Addressing client's individual priorities and keeping clients accountable to themselves are two ways that coaching brings about significant behavior change. Coaches often have their own unique way of approaching a session, which helps them to form a strong rapport with the client and facilitate change.

Since wellness coaches come from a variety of training backgrounds, many different frameworks exist. For example, Wellcoaches, a current leader in the field of wellness coach training, follows a specific framework for initial and follow-up sessions. During an initial session, a client's current lifestyle is assessed. In many corporate programs, a health assessment and the collection of biometrics help the coach and client agree on where the client is now with respect to weight, nutrition, health, exercise, sleep, and level of stress. The coach then assesses a client's readiness to change, a critical element in the coach's ability to meet the client where he is. If the client is ready to change, the coach and client create a wellness vision, a clear picture of where the client wants to go. Once the wellness vision is established, the client identifies the "gap"—the difference between where he is now and where he wants to be, what is motivating him to make the change now, and what might get in the way. This process of developing a vision and uncovering motivators and obstacles leads to the discovery of strategies and eventually to setting long and short-term goals.[3] With the coach's help, clients learn to set goals that are Specific, Measurable, Attainable, Realistic, and Time-bound, otherwise known as SMART goals.[4]

---

[3] Moore, M, ed., Wellcoaches Training Manual. Wellesley, MA: Wellcoaches Corporation; 2004.

[4] Latham, G. 2003. A five step approach to behavior change. Organizational Dynamics. Vol 32 (3) pp. 309-318 (specific page is 311).

Follow-up sessions, which typically occur for approximately three to six months (or until a client meets her goal or goals), are geared toward reviewing the goals from the previous session, discussing victories and challenges, and strategizing how to continue moving towards the long-term goals. It is during these conversations that coaches use their strengths and skills to bring about a generative moment. A generative moment occurs when, through the coach's inquiry, reflection, and support, the client makes a discovery about herself that leads to forward movement.[5]

The coaching approach motivates behavior change because it builds on the client's agenda and is based on key behavioral psychology findings that 1) information alone does not lead to behavior change; rather, people change only when they are motivated to do so and 2) change is facilitated by building on peoples' strengths, rather than highlighting their weaknesses or drawing on fear and guilt as motivators. According to Martin Seligman, founder of positive psychology, "What we attend to, grows."[6] Coaching makes it possible for clients to attend to what's most important to them. It is through this unique relationship that employees truly become empowered to change.

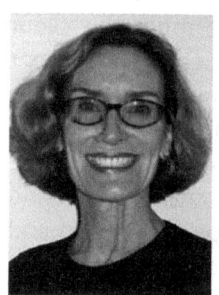 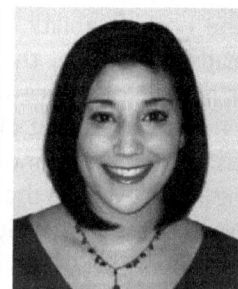

Billie Jo Hance, BS and **Diana Stratigakis**, MAPP, are employed by Take Care Health Systems Employer Solutions, the nation's leading provider of employer-sponsored health, wellness, and fitness and pharmacy programs for large employers. Both authors are Certified Wellness Coaches and Certified Personal Trainers and have helped countless employees improve their health. www.takecarehealth.com

---

[5] Tshannen-Moran B, Jackson E. Generative Moments in Coaching. In: Wellcoaches Training Manual. Wellesley, MA: Wellcoaches Corporation; 2004.
[6] Seligman, Martin E.P. Lecture. Philadelphia, PA. Fall 2005.

Section 3: Occupational Wellness

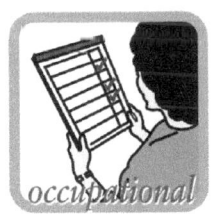

"As I see it every day you do one of two things: build health or produce disease in yourself."

~ Adelle Davis

Section 3: Occupational Wellness

Introduction

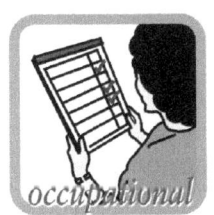

Occupational Wellness focuses on being optimally prepared for the work at hand while gaining personal satisfaction and enrichment. Occupational wellness is achieved by finding the balance between work and leisure knowing its relationship between one's physical and emotional health. It develops the understanding and attitude that decisions and values may change as new information and experiences are attained. It instills flexibility to meet these changes and provides stress management techniques to deal with change in a positive manner.

Characteristics of Occupational Wellness:

- Participating in activities that motivate you personally and professionally
- Engaging in leisure activities that you find enjoyable
- Finding a comfortable direction for future goals and plans
- Understanding personal strengths and weaknesses
- Undertaking what you want to do in life or working toward that goal
- Exhibiting the personal qualities of a valued employee

The Need for Occupational Wellness

Occupational wellness is not optimal within some places of employment. We experience dangerous, demanding, and stressful jobs each day. We feel stressed, pressured, and unfocused leading to poor productivity and job performance. If stress is left untreated, health problems and long-term disease can emerge. Feelings of being "burned out" or overwhelmed have side effects which can include heart attack, depression, diabetes and migraines.

Did you know that ...

- With increasing time spent on the job, job stress is becoming a painful reality for many workers.
- 40% of workers reported that their jobs were very often extremely stressful.
- 25% view their jobs as the number one stressor in their lives.
- 75% of employees believe that they have more on-the-job stress than the generation before them.
- 26% of workers said they were "often or very often burned out or stressed by their work."

Source: Stress At Work by the National Institute for Occupational Safety and Health

- More than one-third of workers say their jobs are harming their physical or emotional health.
- 42% of workers say job pressures are interfering with family and personal relationships.
- 50% of workers say they have a more demanding workload this year than last year.

Source: Attitudes in the American Workplace 8 VII by The Marlin Company.

Occupational Wellness Experts

Occupational Wellness: What is it and how do I achieve it? Learn from **Katy Quinn** the details of occupational wellness including its characteristics and practices. Katy provides questions we can ask ourselves to help steer the course.

Flexibility is key to maintaining health in our workplace. **Janice Newman** gives us eight questions to discover if we are ready to take steps in proposing a flexible work schedule or living up to our end of the bargain in "Are You Ready for Flexible Scheduling?"

Next, "Can That Strong Peppermint Candy Really Help Me to Focus? (The answer: YES!)." Do you sometimes fall asleep at work? Do you sometimes run out of energy during the day? **Nicole**

Pfeffer Crombie explains ways to not only calm but energize us during meetings and throughout the day.

Safe or unsafe. How do we integrate wellness and safety effectively in the workplace? **Jonathan Klane** will show us how to combine the two to improve overall health and safety at work and home.

Finally, **Brian Leonard** looks at "Training your Business: The Proactive vs. Reactive Approach to a Safe Workplace." When the unthinkable happens—Sudden Cardiac Arrest—has our workplace been proactive in preparation or only reacting to the situation in the moment? Brian talks about ways to prepare the workplace for safety and the fundamentals of First Aid Training.

Let's begin!

Occupational Wellness: Personal Assessment

Read the questions and rate yourself from 0 (low level) to 5 (high level) of achievement. Determine the total number for each rating and compare it to the answer key below. This determines where your occupational wellness stands today. Take the test again in 30 days to check your progress on improving occupational wellness. Remember, improvement in any area is *positive action in motion*.

1. I strive to gain professional training to increase my skills and abilities.
    5   4   3   2   1   0

2. I belong to groups and associations that provide me with professional contacts and friendships.
    5   4   3   2   1   0

Occupational Wellness

3. I have written goals and plans for my personal and professional life.

        5   4   3   2   1   0

4. I have learned how to reduce stress on the job.

        5   4   3   2   1   0

5. I manage my time effectively at work.

        5   4   3   2   1   0

6. I have a workload that challenges me but also is manageable.

        5   4   3   2   1   0

7. Most days of the week, I enjoy being at work.

        5   4   3   2   1   0

8. I use my experience and skills to help make my company successful.

        5   4   3   2   1   0

9. I practice the required safety measures on the job.

        5   4   3   2   1   0

10. I exhibit the qualities of an exceptional employee.

        5   4   3   2   1   0

Answer Key: If you answered,

    Mostly **5's** you have an excellent level of occupational wellness. Continue stretching your comfort zone and finding ways to gain greater benefits of being occupationally fit. Consider teaching others how they can reach their occupational wellness goals.

Mostly **4's** you have a high level of occupational wellness. Consider finding innovative ways to make your 4's turn to 5's. This can be fun and exciting.

Mostly **3's** you have a reasonable level of occupational wellness. With a greater attempt and laser focus, you become the model of what it takes to get where you want to be.

Mostly **2's** you're at a good starting point of occupational wellness. Allow yourself to begin again, set goals and go for it!

Mostly **1's** it is time for an upgrade. You have what it takes. Make yourself a priority. Wellness is important to thrive and survive in todays fast pace world.

Mostly **0's** choose one area of occupational wellness to improve upon each month. Seek a buddy to help you find ways to reach your goal, hold you accountable and be your cheerleader. You're worth the investment!

"Treat people as if they were what they ought to be and you help them to become what they are capable of being."
　　　　　　　　　　　　　~ Goethe

Occupational Wellness

Katy D. Quinn, RN, BSN

Occupational Wellness is reflected in the energy we have to put into the job—and the energy we have as we leave the job to pursue the responsibilities and opportunities at the end of our day. It is the resiliency that results from achieving a balance between work and non-work time, and that reflects our ability to address workplace stress and build relationships with co-workers. It requires personal introspection and a compatibility between our career and our personal values, interests, and beliefs. Occupational Wellness recognizes personal satisfaction, gratification, and enrichment in one's life through work.

Occupational Wellness requires healthy adaptation to workplace pressures. Workplace pressures can come from a number of sources:

Relationships

Experiences working with others on teams, committees, and group projects are strongly colored by the relationships of those involved. Creating synergy and satisfaction requires respect and trust among colleagues. Effective teamwork results when members of the team are compatible, bring complementary qualities and talents to the task at hand, and communicate effectively.

Work Demands

The amount of work you need to do, the level of quality that is required, the complexity of the project, the pace at which you need to produce, the meetings that demand your energy, all form your work demands.

Culture and Environment

An open culture where questioning, brainstorming, and risk-taking are practiced and encouraged may be stimulating for some, but threatening for others. Likewise, a highly structured environment with uniform expectations, black and white policies,

Occupational Wellness

strict adherence to procedures and clearly defined roles may be conducive to productivity for some but frighteningly restrictive for others. A culture where personal time is respected may be more conducive to work/family balance, but it may also seem oppressive to the single person who feels discriminated against because she does not have family "excuses" to allow her to leave work early or take time off.

Career Development

When you contribute your unique gifts, skills, and talents to work that is personally meaningful and rewarding, and you receive opportunities to hone those gifts, skills, and talents, you are well on your way to Occupational Wellness. Finding yourself stymied in your current position and without an opportunity to advance creates tremendous workplace pressure, and negatively impacts your Occupational Wellness.

Control of Work

The choice of profession, career ambitions, and personal performance is yours! Those choices are vital to Occupational Wellness. How much control you have over day-to-day tasks can vary. How much control you have over your career path can also vary. If your daily tasks are consistent with your career choice and your personal values, interests, and beliefs as well as your skills and capabilities, and are pointing your career path in a desired direction, your level of Occupational Wellness is likely to be very high. The more inconsistency there is, and the less control you have to influence the compatibility between the demands of the job and your personal preferences and talents, the greater the negative impact on your Occupational Wellness.

Health

How healthy you are in body, mind, emotions, and spirit greatly influences your Occupational Wellness. It is difficult or impossible to work productively if you are ill. On the other hand, being productive is often an antidote for depression—an exciting project can distract us from exhaustion; a sense of accomplishment at work can dull the hurt of personal conflicts. Balance is the key. Moderation is the guide.

Management Practices

If you are someone who needs freedom to create, discover and flourish, a boss who is a micro-manager will debilitate you. If you are a perfectionist who likes to know all the rules and assemble the tools to perform, a boss who leaves it all up to you may make you want to leave. Clear communication—up, down and across the management chain, is conducive to Occupational Wellness. Incentives and rewards that provide the motivation and recognition you crave will make your work days good days. Matching the right manager to the right team contributes greatly to Occupational Wellness.

Individual Characteristics

Who you are and what you care about impact your Occupational Wellness. To help identify your individual characteristics, pause and reflect:

- Where do your passions lie?
- What motivates you? What kind of leadership stimulates you to peak performance?
- What is your fantasy job? What is the ideal occupational opportunity for you?
- Do you prefer a structured environment or a flexible one? Do you like formality or informality?
- How comfortable are you with taking risks?
- What occupations interest you most? What are the favorite jobs you have had?
- Do you prefer working with others on teams or group projects, or do you prefer to work alone?
- Are you most interested in learning through reading and lectures or do you prefer practical and hands-on experience? Or do you thrive with a strong mentor?
- Would you describe yourself as a leader or a follower?
- Add to this list other descriptors of who you are and what is important to you!

Occupational Wellness

The key to Occupational Wellness is having an awareness of what the key sources of our workplace pressures are and which sources of pressure we can do something about. Once we identify the pressure sources that we can influence or change, we can put an action plan in place to optimize our Occupational Wellness.

Pressures create opportunities to stretch! Too much pressure, on the other hand, is detrimental to productivity and to wellness. The trick is to identify and recognize the pressure/performance curve and determine the amount of pressure that brings about growth and excellence without pushing us to the breaking point.

This is similar to interval training in physical fitness, where the athlete pushes herself to discomfort, allows for recovery, and pushes again. As with physical interval training, occupational interval training includes skill building, performance, evaluation, recovery, and persistence.

At the end of the day, check out your Occupational Wellness by asking yourself:

- Am I proud of what I did today?
- Do the good points of my job outweigh the bad ones?
- Am I doing what I want to do with my life?
- Am I a valued and valuable employee?
- Am I comfortable with the direction my life is going and the future I see for my career?
- Are there pressures at work that I can address and change to improve my Occupational Wellness?

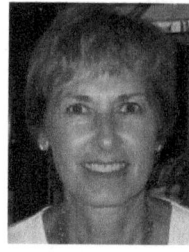

Katy D. Quinn, RN, BSN, is Director of Operations for Take Care Health Systems Employer Solutions, the nation's leading provider of employer-sponsored health, wellness, fitness and pharmacy programs for large employers. Ms. Quinn is a Certified Wellness Coach and has helped numerous companies design and implement successful wellness programs.
www.takecarehealth.com

Are You READY for Flexible Scheduling?
The 8 hard questions you need to ask yourself!

Janice Newman

Setting your own hours.
Working from home.
Taking time off to attend to family or personal issues as they arise.

Flexible scheduling can seem like a "dream come true" for stressed-out employees dealing with demands at home and at work. It's seen as such an important component of employers' recruitment and retention strategies that it is one of the evaluation criteria used to select winners of the Working Mother Magazine's list of 100 Best Companies for Working Mothers. And employers are increasingly viewing flexible scheduling as a necessity to help employees cope with dramatic increases in fuel costs.

You may want to be allowed to set your own hours. Granted, making that happen is largely up to an employer's willingness to do so and up to the parameters and policies already set up in the organization.

So how do policies like this get started?

Mike Foutch, Senior Vice President, Human Resources from First National Bank of Omaha described it this way. "There are always magazines in which you read about the next thing, this is what the best in class is doing, etc." Foutch goes on to say that rather than starting initiatives generated by external sources, the bank redirects, looking internally to the employee population. "We want to be in touch with employees and we listen to them. As we have employees come to us, and they tell us about their jobs and their careers, we listen to what they tell us. They ask about part-time, flex scheduling, and job sharing. It's up to employees to take the initiative and sit down and take the first steps. We are asking employees to step up. And if they do, we listen up!"

Are You READY for Flexible Scheduling?

Kate Martiné, Senior Vice President, Human Resources & Corporate Communications for The Trustmark Companies has a similar approach to flexible scheduling initiatives in the workplace. "Of course we comply with the Family and Medical Leave Act (FMLA) as we should, but it goes much further than that. We need to be sensitive to those family issues, as we all experience them at one time or another in our lives." Martiné has dedicated herself to being creative and finding flexible solutions to help ensure retention of employees in good standing. She went on to say, "We pretty much let people work whatever hours they wish to work as long as it meets the department needs and our external customer needs. I'm not going to simply create some policy or program. I don't believe in policies and rules—rather in guidelines. Then it's up to the employee and to the manager to make it work, which HR will provide assistance with."

So what exactly do all these different terms mean: flexible scheduling, job sharing, etc?

Flexible scheduling at First National Bank of Omaha can mean that instead of the "traditional" 5 x 8 hour days in a workweek, eligible employees can work 3 x 12's or 4 x10's, for example. Foutch gave an additional example of a professional in the audit department who worked nine months and was off 3 months each year.

Martiné described a job sharing initiative at the Trustmark Companies that was suggested by 2 actuaries who were both young women with young families who wanted to stay connected with the workplace, but just couldn't maintain full time working schedules. They suggested combining their two jobs into one and then figured out the "splitting" of job responsibilities. They accepted accountability for achieving performance expectations and took steps to ensure that their internal and external customer service metrics were not only met, but exceeded! Martiné went on to add that there are a lot of employees working 4-day workweeks, especially with so many nurses on staff.

It may sound GREAT to have that kind of freedom, and maybe you and your position are well suited. But maybe your position is not one where there can be this kind of flexibility. And like it or not, maybe you don't have the personality to be able to succeed.

Test yourself by reviewing this 8-point checklist. Your answers will enlighten you on whether you can succeed in this work arrangement.

1. **FIT** – is your position even suitable for flexible scheduling? You may have to accept that it is not. If an organization cannot "mesh" your periodic absences with the organizational goals and commitments to its customers, then it won't happen. The effectiveness of the work relationships while working on a flexible schedule will be paramount. Understand that flexible scheduling is not a right, it's a privilege.

2. **COMMUNICATE** – what are you really trying to achieve? Take a serious look at what you want, why you want it, and how you plan to continue to perform in your job, fully meeting expectations. It's your responsibility to lay out your plan: how you can, and will, continue to provide value and make a contribution.

3. **LIVE UP** to your end of the bargain. Making flexible scheduling work takes a lot including top management buy-in and line manager support. But making it work rests on the employee getting their job done and keeping all promises made during the process of setting up the arrangement.

4. **STAY VISIBLE** – remember the adage "out of sight, out of mind." That was never as appropriate as when discussing flexible scheduling and its potential effect on your career.

5. **BALANCE** can be tough to achieve. Employees typically desire flexible scheduling to help achieve work-life balance. Employers typically provide technology to make flexible scheduling work, such as laptops, PDA's, and cell phones. It's important to be reachable, as you must be available if something happens. But employees sometimes get overwhelmed by being available 24/7 and find themselves constantly distracted, which is exactly the opposite of the desired effect. And similarly, employees working from home sometimes allow themselves to get distracted by the

laundry that has to be done, dinner that should be started, housecleaning, etc., and lose sight of what they are really supposed to be doing, which is focusing on their work.

6. **FLEX** – Employees enjoying flexible scheduling need to be flexible themselves. If you want the organization to flex around your schedule, you need to flex around the organization's schedule. Just because you have been allowed to work a 4-day week does not mean that you are always going to be able to take every Friday off.

7. **RELIEVE** your manager's misgivings, if and when they exist. An organization may be committed to and/or supportive of flexible scheduling but that doesn't mean that your direct supervisor necessarily shares that feeling. A common complaint/concern from managers is that they can't "see" the employee that is telecommuting or working flexible hours. Therefore, that manager doesn't know how to manage that employee effectively because, bluntly said, he/she has no idea if the employee is actually getting their work done. Understand that a manager is ultimately responsible not only for his work, but for the work of all his direct reports. Have a candid conversation with your manager; consider asking him directly if he has these misgivings. Get them out on the table, and get them discussed openly. Then jointly plan and agree on steps that each of you will take to make it work between the two of you.

8. **ADMIT** it when it's not working. Confront it and address it right away. You may be in over your head. You may not be able to exert the self-discipline to get and keep your head in your work, when you know that there is laundry to do, that you have errands to run, or when a favorite TV show is coming on. And when you are sitting in front of your computer, you may find yourself getting constantly distracted by personal emails or surfing the internet. Self-discipline is absolutely critical to making this work. If you find that you are falling into a trap of never seeming to be able to focus on work, then sit yourself down and ask yourself the hard questions to see if you are cut out for flexible scheduling. Maybe you're not and the more

traditional work schedule, coming in to the brick-and-mortar office, is better for you. Don't wait to see if your manager "figures out" that you are not being productive; make an appointment with him and talk about transitioning back out of flexible scheduling.

Ask yourself these hard questions. Be critical of your own answers. Talk at length with the stakeholders in your personal life. Write a well thought out objective and create your plan on how you will make this work. Come up with performance metrics, how you will meet them, and how often you will measure yourself. Make an appointment with your supervisor and/or HR (depending on how your organization handles requests like these).

You may very well be the next employee at your organization to enjoy the privilege of flexible scheduling!

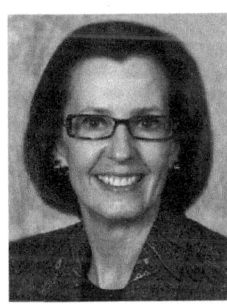

Janice Newman earned her MBA and a MHRM (Masters' in Human Resources Management) from Keller Graduate School in Chicago. In addition, she has a Senior Professional in Human Resources (SPHR) certification from the Human Resource Certification Institute and is a Certified Employment Law Specialist (CELS) from Columbia Southern University. www.hrfocusco.com

> "The... patient should be made to understand that he or she must take charge of his own life. Don't take your body to the doctor as if he were a repair shop."
> ~ Quentin Regestein

Can that Strong Peppermint Candy Really Help Me to Focus? (The Answer: YES!)

Nicole Pfeffer Crombie

Do you ever get stressed out at work? Or do you ever feel like you're going to fall asleep at work? If you answered yes to one (or both) of these questions, you are not alone! Picture this scenario: You have a deadline for work that is fast approaching and you have been procrastinating until now. You figured you could pull it off in a day or so but you are quickly realizing that it is going to require a lot more of your time and energy than you originally thought. As you start the project, you quickly become overwhelmed and start to panic as you think of how soon the deadline is approaching and how little you have actually prepared. I would be willing to say that your heart is probably beating a little faster than it normally does, your palms are sweatier than usual, and you really feel like you want to scream and bail out. Right now, you are experiencing a state of over-stimulation. Other terms that might be a little more familiar to you are feeling "anxious," "on edge," or "stressed out."

In contrast, have you ever felt like you were going to fall asleep at work? Now picture this scenario: the company has called a meeting that everyone must attend. The meeting is a presentation on a subject that you are not particularly interested in. Everyone is sitting around the table with their heads in their hands. The air is very warm. The speaker is incredibly boring and speaks with a monotone voice. The light is dimmed while the video presentation is on the screen and people are starting to nod off (including you). How are you feeling right now? You are probably feeling a slow pulse rate, your breathing is slow and steady, and you just want to rest your head on your arms. In fact, I bet you could fall asleep just thinking about it! Right now, you are experiencing a state of under-stimulation. Other words you may have used to describe this state are "lethargic", "bored", or "lazy."

You are not going to be productive when you are so stressed out that you cannot think straight let alone perform your job duties. You are also not going to be productive when you are so bored out of your mind that you are ready to fall asleep on the table. Neither one of these states is conducive to working productively. In order to be at your maximal potential at work, you should be at a "neutral" level, meaning that you are not feeling "stressed out" or "lethargic." I am an occupational therapist working in the school system. Occupational therapists often use what we call a "sensory diet" or other programs for the students that help them to regulate themselves (either to calm or to alert themselves). One wonderful program we teach is called "How Does Your Engine Run" and it has helped students to regulate themselves at school based on a simple concept of an engine and feeling "just right." This concept of alerting and calming can be used to help achieve that "just right" feeling at work as well. You really do need a neutral feeling (meaning not feeling bored or not feeling anxious) to work well and to be productive while working. You are probably asking, "What can I do while I am working to achieve that 'just right' feeling in order to be more productive?"

There are some really simple things that you can do on a regular basis to help you achieve that "neutral" or "just right" level. By changing some things within your sensory environment—through your eyes, mouth, skin, ears, nose, and/or muscles—you can quickly change your level of alertness without taking great measures that disrupt everyone in the work environment (such as becoming frustrated with the noise level, picking up all of your materials, frantically moving to a different space, loudly dropping the pile onto a new table, and in return disrupting all of your co-workers). In the following lists, I give examples of what you can do to help you calm or energize yourself to achieve that optimal level of productivity. I have also categorized the examples into the appropriate sensory subcategories. Some examples that I include may appear in both the "calming" and "energizing" sections. This is not a typo. These activities are unique in that they do both—calm and energize—depending on where you are functioning at the time!

To Calm Your:

Eyes:
- Decrease the intensity of the lights (or close the blinds)
- Look at warm colors (browns, tans, etc.)

- Clean your workspace to decrease the clutter
- Look at a joke or a funny picture as a break
- Take a break to look at something soothing such as a picture of your loved one/s, a picture of the beach/ocean, etc.

Mouth:
- Chew something hard such as bubblegum, beef jerky, licorice, or fruit snacks
- Use a straw to drink something
- Eat crunchy items such as peanuts, pretzels, carrots, or celery
- Suck on a piece of candy that has a soothing flavor such as vanilla or butterscotch
- Drink something warm such as hot tea

Skin:
- Squeeze a stress ball (or a fidget toy such as a rubber band ball)
- Increase the temperature of the room

Ears:
- Listen to slow music using headphones or your iPod (quietly)
- Use earplugs in your ears to drown out extraneous noise in the environment

Nose:
- Smell the calming scents of lavender or vanilla (using a plug diffuser as needed, an air freshener kept in your drawer, or use essential oils on cotton balls)

Muscles:
- Perform chair push-ups (place hands on your seat; push up with your hands/arms)
- Shift your weight in your seat

Can that Peppermint Candy Really Help Me to Focus?

- Press the palms of your hands together
- Roll your shoulders back and forth
- Stretch at your desk
- Take a walk outside in the natural sunlight
- Take a walk up the stairs
- Work-out on your lunch break
- Take deep breaths
- Carry something heavy (such as a stack of books) to another location

To Energize Your:

Eyes:
- Increase the lighting in the area (open the blinds or add a lamp if necessary)
- Take a walk outside in the natural sunlight
- Look at vibrant colors (hot pink, yellow, etc.)
- Look at a joke or a funny picture as a break
- Look at a picture that energizes you as a break (can be anything…a picture of your favorite rock band performing?)

Mouth:
- Chew gum or other food item that requires energy (such as beef jerky, licorice, bubble gum, etc.)
- Suck on a piece of candy with a strong flavor such as peppermint or orange
- Drink something cold (such as cold bottled water with lemon juice)
- Eat something that is either: sour (pickles), salty (salted peanuts, popcorn), or spicy (salsa, beef jerky); these all increase your alert levels
- Eat crunchy food items such as carrots, pretzels, celery, cucumbers, etc.

Skin:
- Use a fidget toy such as a squeeze ball, rubber band ball, etc.
- Decrease the temperature of the room (or add a fan if necessary)

Ears:
- Listen to fast music with headphones (loudly to really get the effect)

Nose:
- Smell the strong scents of peppermint, lemon, or grapefruit using essential oils, plug-ins, etc.

Muscles:
- Take a walk up the stairs or outside
- Work-out on your lunch break
- Do chair push-ups
- Shift your weight in your seat
- Press the palms of your hands together
- Roll your shoulders back and forth
- Stretch at your desk
- Take deep breaths
- Carry something heavy (such as a stack of books) to another location

There are many things that you can do using your sensory systems throughout the workday to increase your concentration levels and therefore help to increase your productivity. These are ideas that you can use on a daily basis for yourself that will not disrupt your co-workers. In addition, they need not apply only to the work environment—you can use these to help you in your home environment as well. Whether you are feeling anxious (in which case you may choose to drink some warm tea) or sluggish (in which case you may pop one of those strong peppermint candies), you have the ability to change your stimulation levels and be more productive in the workforce and in your own life.

Can that Peppermint Candy Really Help Me to Focus?

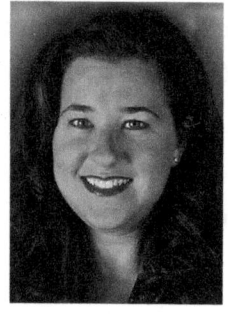

Nicole Pfeffer Crombie received her bachelor's degree from Allegheny College in Meadville, PA and her master's degree in occupational therapy from Chatham University in Pittsburgh, PA. She has worked in outpatient pediatric rehab, the school systems, and early intervention/home care. She currently resides in Charlottesville, VA with her family and works in the school system of Virginia. ncrombie@comcast.net.

Combine Wellness with Workplace Safety and Health
12 Steps You Can Take to Increase Your Total Health!

Jonathan Klane, M.S.Ed., CIH, CHMM, CET

Both wellness and workplace occupational health and safety (OHS) have benefits to employees and employers alike. While both can be implemented separately, there are proven additional benefits to combining the two programs into one overall Employee Health, Safety, and Wellness (HSW) Program where the total is greater than the sum of the parts. Combine your efforts in these 12 areas and enjoy improved wellness.

Readers will gain a list of areas to combine, where to start, and most importantly, improved wellness by following the tips in these areas. As you read, here are some considerations to help you focus:

- Which wellness or health issues do I face?
- Which OHS areas does my company face?
- What can I do to improve my total health?
- How can I get help from my company?
- What will I use as my "yardstick" to measure my progress?

Let's start with areas where this works. Here are a dozen aspects of OHS where combining wellness just makes perfect sense.

1. **Obesity and ergonomics/cancers**: Studies show that persons who are overweight or obese (O/O) are more likely to have ergonomics problems[1] and are more likely to have greater worker compensation claims.[2] Also, persons

---

[1] Kort, M. and Baldry, J., "The association between musculoskeletal disorders and obesity." Australian Health Review, 2002;25(6):207-14.

[2] "Obesity Increases Workers' Compensation Costs", Duke Medicine News and Communications, April 23, 2007.

who are O/O are more likely to get cancer including breast, colon, lung, prostate, and others.[3] Dump the pounds and lower your cancer and ergonomics risks. Ask your OHS person about workplace and home ergonomics and carcinogens.

2. **Smoking and ergonomics, carbon monoxide, and asbestos:** Studies have shown that smokers tend to have more ergonomics problems.[4] Smokers also have higher levels of carbon monoxide (CO) gas in their blood. This puts smokers at greater risk of CO poisoning depending blood level.[5] OSHA Region I (the northeast) investigated a fatality many years ago where a worker died of CO poisoning from a combination of 3 sources: CO from fork trucks, CO from smoking, and CO (in their blood) from methylene chloride (MeCl) exposure. MeCl (a common ingredient of paint strippers) metabolizes in the body into CO. None of the three sources individually was enough to be fatal; however, the combination of all three was enough.[6] Smokers are 50–92 times more likely to get lung cancer from asbestos than non-smokers. Stop smoking to cut your risk of dying from other causes (in addition to tobacco). Ask your OHS person about ergonomics (again), CO, MeCl, and asbestos exposures at work.

3. **Fitness and ergonomics:** Fitness level and ergonomics are related—as one goes up, the other goes down (and vice versa).[7] Since fitness counts, ask your OHS person about advice on strength and flexibility training—join a gym, take up yoga, do cardio.

---

[3] "Obesity and Cancer: Questions and Answers", National Cancer Institute, March 16, 2004.

[4] Jain, Vijay Kumar, "Smoking Related Musculoskeletal Disorders – A Review", Journal of Orthopaedics, 2006.

[5] Nordenberg, D., Yip, R., Binki, N.J., "The effect of cigarette smoking on hemoglobin levels and anemia screening", Journal of the American Medical Association, Volume 264, Number 12, Sept. 26, 1990.

[6] Interview with Douglas Lawson, Ph.D., CIH, former OSHA Compliance Officer Region 1.

[7] NIOSH Publication 97-141, "A Critical Review of Epidemiologic Evidence for Work-Related MSDs of the Neck, Upper Extremity, and Low Back", June 1997.

4. **Job activity level and prostate cancer:** Job activity level and prostate cancer are also related (as one goes up, the other goes down).[8] So, men need to be more active in their jobs to cut prostate cancer risk. Ask your OHS person about increasing your activity level. Get up and walk around more if you work in an office. Take the stairs. Park farther away. Lots of little activities add up and do make a difference.

5. **Exposures off and on the job—asbestos, CO, solvents, acids/bases, sensitizers, lead:** It's pretty obvious. There are many chemicals and other hazardous substances that you can be exposed to at home and off the job. Asbestos in older homes, CO from our vehicles (and other combustion sources), solvents in cleaners and degreasers, acids and bases in cleaners—the list goes on and on. Ask your OHS person about products you use at home and what you should do to avoid exposures.

6. **Healthy foods at work and obesity and cancers:** We eat at least one meal at work, often two, and sometimes even all three meals in a day. Nutritional needs are at least one-half of the O/O problem in the U.S. We tend to eat whatever is readily available to us regardless of its nutritional value or our willpower. O/O is linked to several cancers and other chronic and costly health issues (diabetes, metabolic syndrome, heart disease, etc.). Ask your company about healthy options in the cafeteria, vending machines, etc.

7. **Driving safety:** Without even counting fatal accidents during normal work commutes, driving is the leading cause of work-related fatalities.[9] 9 Whatever we can do to drive safer the better. Ask your OHS person about safe driving training at work.

8. **Genetic link to diseases and target organs of chemicals:** There is a great saying, "Your genes load the

---

[8] Krishnadasan, Anusha, Dr. et. al., University of California, Los Angeles, *Cancer Causes Control*, Feb. 2008.

[9] NIOSH Publication No. 2003-119: Work-Related Roadway Crashes - Challenges and Opportunities for Prevention, Sept. 2003.

gun—the environment pulls the trigger." For many of us the gun is already loaded. We have heart disease, high blood pressure, various cancers, etc. in our gene pool and so it's even more important for us to avoid environmental factors that are linked to those diseases. Some environmental triggers are the chemicals and other hazardous substances we're exposed to at work and off the job. Chemicals typically "target" certain organs—they cause damage to specific organs. These "target organs" vary among chemicals. Some examples include asbestos, silica, and many mineral dusts that target the lungs and respiratory system. Acetone and other solvents target the brain, central nervous system (CNS), skin, etc. Methylene chloride is linked to the blood system and the liver (causing cancer). Benzene is also linked to the blood system and causes leukemia. Lead has many target organs including the brain and CNS, heart, kidneys, liver, and reproductive system (making it a "teratogen"). Ask your OHS person about chemicals and target organs. Look for this information on material safety data sheets (MSDSs), too.

9. **Stress:** Work-related stress is a common factor in employee surveys and complaints. The effects of stress of the body are many and varied. These include mental health, obesity, the gastrointestinal system, heart, endocrine system, tooth and gum disease, and diabetes to name a few.[10] Reducing stress (both at home and at work) is an obvious way to reduce health problems and complaints. Worker complaints about stress are often tied to a lack of control over their work and workload. If you're feeling stressed out (at work or home), ask about your company's employee assistance plan (EAP).

10. **Home safety and work safety:** More accidents occur off the job than on the job—and that's just to workers (it does not include non-workers, e.g. children and the elderly or infirmed). These accidents account for 25% more lost time than on the job accidents, too.[11] Focusing solely on work-

---

[10] NIOSH Publication No. 99-101: "STRESS...At Work", 1999.
[11] University of Alaska Fairbanks, Safety Sentinel, 2000.

related accidents is getting at less than half of the problem and causes. Ask your OHS person about home safety.

11. **Behavior-based safety and lifestyle changes:** We are such creatures of habit and many of us would attest to the cliché "old habits are hard to break." Whether they are safety-related habits at work (wearing my respirator) or personal health-related habits (eating a lot of fried foods) they impact our overall health and safety. Talk to your OHS person about safe behaviors at work and home.

12. **Urban myths/internet hoaxes:** We all get them—an email that warns us of some unknown hazard and implores us to forward it immediately to everyone in our address book. Of course we also get them at our homes from well meaning friends. The next time you get one, check it out first (before forwarding it) at www.snopes.com or other urban legend sites. Ask your OHS person about these when you get them.

Certainly there are other areas where combining wellness with workplace safety makes sense. More studies will undoubtedly continue to demonstrate the overlap between work and home life and the obvious benefits of combining the two together. For now, focus your energies on these 12 tips to workplace (and personal) wellness. Be well!

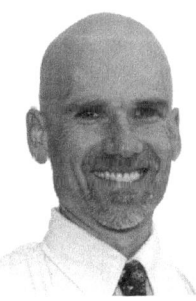

Jonathan Klane, M.S.Ed., CIH, CHMM, CET provides health, safety, training, wellness, and consulting services and is a faculty member at Thomas College in their Graduate Program teaching EHS and Wellness. He is a seasoned conference presenter, author and developer of on-line Webinars on Training, Wellness, and Health and Safety topics. Contact him at jonathan@trainerman.com
www.trainerman.com

"We now have unshakable conviction that accident causes are man-made and that a manmade problem can be solved by men and women."
    ~ *W.H. Cameron*

Training your Business: The Proactive vs. Reactive Approach to a Safe Workplace

Brian Leonard

If you were to ask most company CEOs in the United States for a list of their top five concerns for their businesses, there is little doubt that employee safety would rank high on that list. However, most companies do not pay enough attention to this issue until after a workplace fatality has occurred. This leaves the company dealing with massive personal and monetary losses that could have easily been prevented with the right training and foresight.

The most important training that a company can implement is training its management to think proactively when it comes to employee safety. Put in monetary terms, the numbers are simply staggering. In 2004 alone, there were an estimated 4.3 million work-related injuries and illnesses and of those, 5,703 were fatal. The average cost to employers just for one on-site fatality cost close to one million dollars. Now, keep in mind that does not factor in the cost of occupational illnesses and injuries which, combined with the cost of fatalities, can amount to a 143 billion dollar burden for the United States economy.[1]

One of the most preventable workplace fatalities is Sudden Cardiac Arrest (SCA). If an employee suffers from SCA in the workplace and does not receive prompt and effective care, the employee may die.[2] Perhaps the most unsettling fact is that some of this nation's largest cities have such low survival rates for SCA. For example, Chicago has one of the lowest in the country—only two percent. What makes this so frustrating is that when a workplace takes the proactive approach and implements a First-Aid program, not only does the survival rate increase, but the cost to the employer decreases. The program can ultimately be the difference between life and death.

---

[1] National Safety Council. (2006). *Injury Facts*, 2004-2006 Edition. Itasca, IL pg. 51
[2] Occupational Safety and Health Administration

Training your Business:
The Proactive vs. Reactive Approach to a Safe Workplace

There are several simple steps that should be taken to proactively train a workplace in the fundamentals of First Aid. First, the company should make an effort to obtain EMS response times for all business locations during all days and times of operation. This will allow for the company, as well as employees, to be aware of how long it will take for emergency support to arrive on the scene. Second is determining the need for CPR training and automated external defibrillator (AED) needs. With all of the recent advances in technology, AEDs are now readily available for use in the workplace and are extremely user-friendly. They provide critical treatment for SCA and can boost the survival rate to over 60%.[3] For those who are unfamiliar with the benefits of CPR training and the exact purpose of an AED, the basic benefits are that CPR supports circulation and ventilation until the electric shock administered by an AED can restore the heart to normal fibrillating rhythms. This can ultimately be the difference between life and death, which can translate directly to the amount of money that a company risks losing due to a workplace fatality.

The final steps to creating a First Aid program in the workplace are site assessment, educating employees on the crucial steps that should be taken in an emergency, executing national training and AED implementation and finally, AED program management to keep in compliance with evolving regulations.

Employers should begin to look for and utilize safe measures and proper tools so those can be available in case of an emergency. Businesses can feel overwhelmed by the thought of implementing a First Aid program and as a direct result postpone enlisting someone to administer the proper training. First Aid programs should be crafted to specifically cater to each individual company. What works for one may not work for another. That is why site assessment is critical. There are companies who have made it their mission to reach out to businesses of all sizes and help them focus on these critical steps. Our company, Code Red helps companies and communities alike to take the proactive approach to

---

[3] American Heart Association in collaboration with International Liaison Committee on Resurrection. Guidelines 200 for Cardiopulmonary Resuscitation and Emergency Cardiovascular Care: International Consensus on Science, Part 4: The Automated External Defibrillator. Circulation. 2000; Vol. 102, Supplement: I 61. Figure1.

preventing workplace fatalities by giving them the correct tools to anticipate the risks of their working environment. That, partnered with site maintenance, employee training, and the relevant tools such as AED devices, raises survival rates after something such as SCA occurs.

Having up-to-date AED devices that employees feel safe using and arming them with knowledge of the correct protocol to follow in the event of an on-site emergency are necessary to having a confident and safe staff. By implementing proactive employee safety programs companies show that they are genuinely concerned about their well-being.

Brian Leonard is the President and CEO of Code Red, LLC. Code Red addresses the need for workplace safety by creating emergency response teams, implementing AEDs, as well as CPR and first aid training programs. Code Red provides national CPR/First Aid/AED programs and management for many Fortune 500 corporations. Brian is on the board for the GMA division of the American Heart Association, National Advisory Committee for Alzheimer's foundation, Committee member National Association of EMS Educators education committee, and a member of the president's circle for the Chicagoland Chamber of Commerce.   www.coderedcpr.com

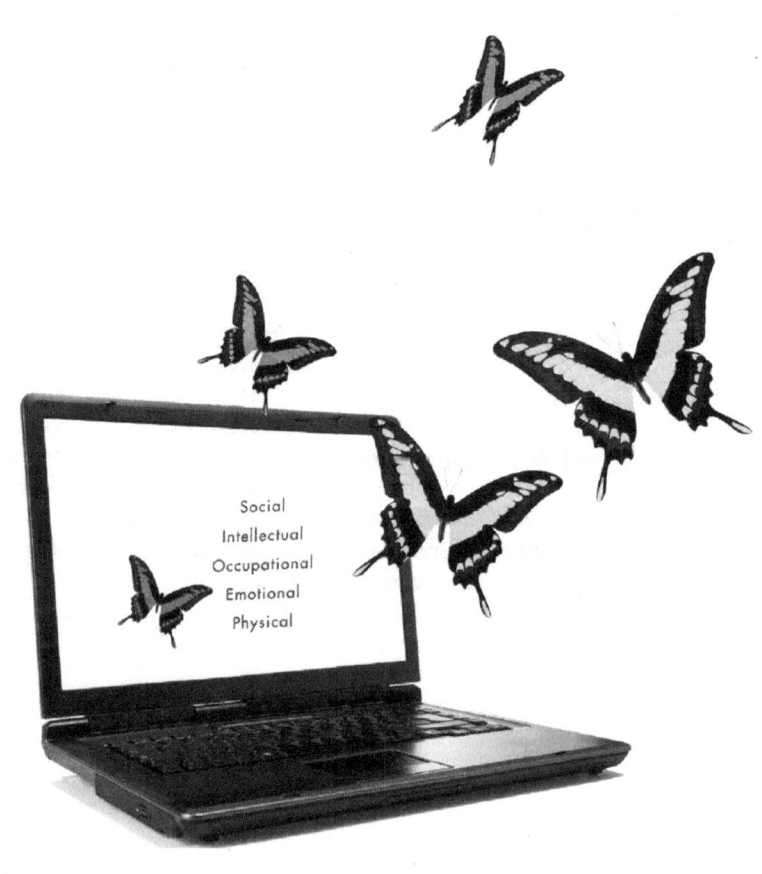

Section 4: Emotional Wellness

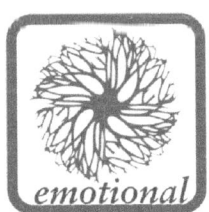

"Let's not forget that the little emotions are the great captains of our lives and we obey them without realizing it."
           ~Vincent Van Gogh, 1889

Section 4: Emotional Wellness

Introduction

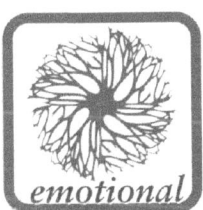

Emotional Wellness is the ability to recognize and understand a wide range of feelings in ourselves and others. It is being able to freely express and manage one's own feelings to develop a positive self-image and to arrive at personal decisions based on attitudes and behaviors. Emotional wellness is achieved by continually working on positive self-esteem, relationships that are rich in satisfaction, and learning to meet life's challenges with resilience.

Characteristics of Emotional Wellness:
- Self confidence in our abilities and talents
- Self acceptance
- Recognizing our problems
- Ability to find solutions for problems and issues
- Coping through challenges in healthy ways
- Managing our feelings and emotions

Our emotional well-being can be compared to circus juggling. When all is going smoothly, the areas of our life are juggled with ease, creating synergy and stability. When life events tip our emotions, these same areas can get out of sync and life appears unbalanced. Emotions such as anger, worry, and grief are a part of life. When one or more of these begin to consume our thoughts and our days, they can damage our personal relationships with friends and family as well as seriously hurt our professional associations.

Emotional Wellness

The Need for Emotional Wellness

Edward Hallowell writes that modern office life is turning steady executives into frenzied underachievers:

"[This] experience is becoming the norm for overworked managers who suffer—like many of your colleagues, and possibly like you—from a very real but unrecognized neurological phenomenon that I call attention deficit trait, or ADT. Caused by brain overload,

ADT is now epidemic in organizations. The core symptoms are distractibility, inner frenzy, and impatience.

"I have observed firsthand how a rapidly growing segment of the adult population is developing this ... condition. The number of people with ADT coming into my clinical practice has mushroomed by a factor of ten in the past decade.

"Blessed with the largest cortex in all of nature, owners of this trillion-celled organ today put singular pressure on the frontal and prefrontal lobes [which] guide decision making and planning. ... As long as our frontal lobes remain in charge, everything is fine.

"Beneath the frontal lobes lie the parts of the brain devoted to survival. These deep centers govern basic functions ... as well as crudely positive and negative emotions. When you are doing well and operating at peak level, the deep centers send up messages of excitement, satisfaction, and joy. They pump up your motivation, help you maintain attention, and don't interfere with working memory, the number of data points you can keep track of at once. But when you are confronted with the sixth decision after the fifth interruption in the midst of a search for the ninth missing piece of information on the day that the third deal has collapsed and the 12th impossible request has blipped unbidden across your computer screen, your brain begins to panic, reacting just as if that sixth decision were a bloodthirsty, man-eating tiger.

"Intelligence dims. In a futile attempt to do more than is possible, the brain paradoxically reduces its ability to think clearly."

Overloaded Circuits: Why Smart People Underperform,
Edward M. Hallowell, Harvard Business Review January 2005

Did you know? ...

Emotional wellness is revealed by the acceptance of a full range of feelings from positive emotions such as happiness, excitement, contentment, and love contribute to an overall sense of well-being. We can meet emotional needs constructively and maintain a positive attitude, high self-esteem, and a strong self-image. When we are in touch with our range of emotions, we stand a greater chance of leading a healthy life.

Emotional Wellness Experts

Join **Dr. Arien van der Merwe** as she explains that it's not impossible to head towards "Going for the Gold – Maintaining Work-Life Balance." Work-life balance has become an increasingly sought after topic as we try to do and be it all at the same time. Learn that it starts with you and how to manage your highest priority.

We also need to forgive ourselves as the starting point. **Retta Flagg** talks about the forgiveness process and why it's necessary in all human relations in "To Err Is Human –To Forgive Is Healthy."

As **Patrice Rancour** writes, "The post-modern world is a stressful place." In her article, "Emotional Wellness: Keeping It Real and Keeping Your Cool, When All Around You, Others are Losing Theirs," learn techniques to reduce stress and be in control.

Finally, when loss at the workplace comes in the form of job, people or projects, how do we effectively cope? **Dr. Kirsti Dyer** explains in, "Loss and the Workplace: What to Do at Work When the World Crashes in Around You," the different types of workplace loss and suggestions for helping ourselves and others move towards a positive outlook.

Let's begin!

Emotional Wellness

Emotional Wellness: Personal Assessment

Read the questions and rate yourself from 0 (low level) to 5 (high level) of achievement. Determine the total number for each rating and compare it to the answer key below. This determines where your emotional wellness stands today. Take the test again in 30 days to check your progress on improving emotional wellness. Remember, improvement in any area is *positive action in motion*.

1. I have more positive relationships than negative ones.
   5   4   3   2   1   0

2. I'm working on decreasing clutter in my home, office, and car.
   5   4   3   2   1   0

3. I'm able to work through conflict, reaching a win-win ending.
   5   4   3   2   1   0

4. I don't take work issues personally.
   5   4   3   2   1   0

5. I feel good about who I am and where I'm going.
   5   4   3   2   1   0

6. I have an adequate level of work/life balance.
   5   4   3   2   1   0

7. I set boundaries around my life to reduce over-commitment.
   5   4   3   2   1   0

8. I regularly practice ways to reduce stress.

        5   4   3   2   1   0

9. I see change as opportunities to personally and professionally grow.

        5   4   3   2   1   0

10. I deal with only the facts of situations to reduce emotional decisions.

        5   4   3   2   1   0

Answer Key: If you answered,

Mostly **5's** you have an excellent level of emotional wellness. Continue stretching your comfort zone and finding ways to gain greater benefits of being emotionally fit. Consider teaching others how they can reach their emotional wellness goals.

Mostly **4's** you have a high level of emotional wellness. Consider finding innovative ways to make your 4's turn to 5's. This can be fun and exciting.

Mostly **3's** you have a reasonable level of emotional wellness. With a greater attempt and laser focus, you become the model of what it takes to get where you want to be.

Mostly **2's** you're at a good starting point of emotional wellness. Allow yourself to begin again, set goals and go for it!

Mostly **1's** it's time for an upgrade. You have what it takes. Make yourself a priority. Wellness is important to thrive and survive in todays fast pace world.

Mostly **0's** choose one area of emotional wellness to improve upon each month. Seek a buddy to help you find ways to reach your goal, hold you accountable and be your cheerleader. You're worth the investment!

"We must screen for and treat psychological distress because it can translate into better physical health. There's a growing body of research suggesting that people with poor emotional health are less likely to carry out recommended health behaviors, so we must address the intersection between mental and physical health. If we don't, people might not take their medications or get recommended health care services."
~ *Joshua Thorpe, Ph.D., MPH*
Duke University Center for Aging

Going for the Gold
Maintaining Work-Life Balance

Dr. Arien van der Merwe, MBChB, FRIPH, FRCAM, MISMA

Stress can be positive or negative. When stress sparks personal achievement or life enjoyment and appreciation (positive stress), it can work to your benefit by making you enthusiastic, creative and productive, motivating you. But stress can easily spiral out of control, becoming negative distress, taking its toll on your physical and emotional health and well-being if you don't carefully balance all aspects of your life: work, relationships including family and friends, personal growth, playtime, and fun.

Stress is not an illness, but it can lead to specific physical and emotional symptoms, often serious enough to send people to the emergency room or their health care practitioner's office. According to the American Psychological Association, 43% of adults suffer adverse health effects from stress, and 75–90% of all visits to a doctor are stress related. Women are experiencing more stress at every stage of their lives than ever before. Juggling professional life, education needs, family schedules, money issues, career advancement, child- and elder-care concerns are only a few of the common stress triggers confronting women.

What is work-life balance?

It's the eternal striving for balance between work and the rest of your life. Is 100% balance possible? No! But you can try to the best of your ability to get as close to perfect balance as possible. The top stress workplace health challenge complaints are family or marital problems, deadlines, work-related stress, fatigue, and a sense that life seems unsatisfactory and unbalanced, sort of "is this all there is?" Of course, these are often closely related. We simply feel that there's never enough time and energy, or we don't know what to do to "fix" things. Short of having oneself cloned, something's bound to draw the shortest end of the stick. Usually it's personal or family life. Work is the easy winner. The good news is that radical lifestyle changes aren't required. Standing back, trying to see the bigger picture, then making one or two small, personally strategic changes, are often all that's necessary.

Why do we need this balance?

If we consider the dimensions of our ideal lives, we have to include the physical body, the mental body or intellect (related to left brain function), the emotional body (related to the limbic system and right side of the brain), the soul body (related to life meaning & purpose, also right brain function), the occupational or work dimension; the social dimension of interaction with others and groups and also the environmental dimension, where we form part of a bigger picture, from communities, to the natural, global and universal environment. To remain in balance—healthy, happy and joyfully alive—we have to allocate enough time to each of these dimensions. As soon as one is out of balance, the scale tips and we become unbalanced energy conductors.

Stress can cause a variety of physical ailments, from headache to symptoms that mimic a heart attack. In addition, stress can cause depression and anxiety. Stress might even trigger illness, such as high blood pressure, high cholesterol, diabetes mellitus, eczema, irritable bowel syndrome, severe menopausal symptoms, and asthma.

One-minute stress busters

Breathe in deeply through your nose on a slow count of three. Push your stomach out as you breathe in. Hold it for a count of three. Breathe out through your mouth on a slow count of six. Repeat two or more times. Try this every time you feel stressed, anxious, or worried. Do it every morning before you get up and every night before falling asleep. Feel your pulse rate by putting your fingers gently on your wrist below the thumb. When you're stressed, it's fast. Do the slow breathing and feel how your pulse rate slows down—a quick fix stress buster!

Tired eye soother

Splash eyes with cold water; alternate with a hot washcloth over your closed eyelids and press gently with your fingertips.

Rub an ice cube around each eye.

Lie back in your chair or on a bed, place sliced cucumber or a wet tea bag over your closed eyes and relax for a few minutes.

Do eye exercises: blink a few times, focus on objects far and then near, move your eyes in a circle while keeping your head still, rub the palms of your hands vigorously together and place over your closed eyelids.

Support your body for internal balance

Have regular mini-breaks every 2 hours from sitting or standing where your muscles remain in one position all the time. Breathe deeply, get up and stretch your neck, arms and shoulders, roll your shoulders clockwise and counterclockwise, clasp your hands behind your back and lift your arms, shake your legs, drink herbal tea, look out the window. This will prevent tension headaches and neck muscle spasm.

Exercise regularly. Find something you enjoy. Nia technique dance, yoga, Tai 'chi, Pilates, Powerplate exercises, belly dancing, modern dancing, are all different and enjoyable activities to try. The wellness definition of physical fitness is to obtain and maintain the ability to meet the needs of your lifestyle with ease.

Balancing food tips

- **Prevent low blood sugar**—it's a stress attractor! Eat regular, healthy, small meals. Always have fruit, veggies, nuts and seeds handy!
- **Sip away your stress:** chamomile, mint, passionflower, lemon balm, ginseng, lavender, valerian herbal teas, together with a spoonful of honey will soothe frazzled nerves.
- **Calming foods:** tryptophane boosts the formation of serotonin, the "feel good," calming brain chemical—eat unrefined carbohydrates, nuts and bananas.
- **Energizing foods:** small amounts of protein (cheese, eggs, chicken, meat) contain the amino acid tryptamine that can give you a boost when stress tires you out. Take small ready-prepared portions to work.
- **Take a daily dose of vitamin B-complex** to support your nervous system together with an antioxidant and

multivitamin combination (vitamin A, E, C, minerals zinc, selenium, copper, chromium, iron, calcium and magnesium).
- **Use the herb Ginkgo biloba** to boost your concentration and memory.
- **Food for thought:** beans / legumes, lean meat, whole grain and enriched cereals, poultry, fish such as trout, salmon, tuna, sardines and mackerel, dairy products, brewer's yeast, nuts, seeds, fruit, vegetables.

Listen to music to help you balance your mood: uplifting with a beat to increase your energy when it's low or you're feeling down; slow and flowing when you feel overwhelmed by stress emotions like anger, fear, worry, anxiety.

Include balancing tools in your workplace

Take regular breathing and mini-breaks: breathe deeply and slowly for 2 minutes every 2 hours, drink a calming and relaxing herbal tea (e.g. lavender, chamomile, orange blossom, hibiscus blends) while really bringing mindful attention to the smell, taste and experience of drinking the tea. Use your lunch break to take a walk in a nearby park. Arrange a small chill room at work where you can sit back, relax, and listen to soothing music for a few minutes. Have plants and fresh flowers in your office. Use pictures or photographs as focus points for mindfulness.

Manage techno stress by looking at the ergonomics of your computer screen, keyboard, chair, fresh air circulation, and sufficient natural light. Take a break outside for fresh air therapy! Prevent information overload by taking week-end techno breaks: cell phones off, laptops hidden from view, don't watch the news. Learn to switch off, unwind, and relax. Go out in nature to establish a link with the earth.

Relationships for balance: make enough time for family and friends to comply with the social dimension needed for human health and happiness.

All relationships start by first having a relationship with yourself:
- Use positive self-talk and affirmations to remove doubt, fear, and worry.
- Actively cultivate a sense of humor by watching comedies, reading joke books, laughing with your partner, family, and friends.
- Know your own values, goals, and priorities.
- Be assertive—learn how to ask for what you want or need.
- Set boundaries. We often allow loved ones to stretch us far beyond our limits because we find it harder to say no to kids or partner. It's important to make time for family, but also to make time for your physical, mental & spiritual health.

Maintain relationship with others for social balance:
- Build and maintain support systems by using the tend-and-befriend response.
- Invest in relationships with your spouse / partner, kids, friends, family, community, pets.
- Clear communication is the key to successful relationships.
- Intimacy develops though frequent contact and connection with others.

Ensure daily quiet time for balance and integration of right and left brain. Remember, we are human beings, not human doings! Take time out every day to sit quietly and reflect. To experience nature: it is your root. Become aware of your own breath: it is the source of your energy.

Manage your life away from work through creativity and hobbies (kids and partner can join for quality family time!). Make time for play, joy, laughter, and fun.

Always dig deep inside your own soul to find your life's meaning and purpose by asking the following questions:
- Who am I?

- Why am I here?
- Am I fulfilling my purpose?
- What are my values and beliefs?
- What is the meaning of my life?

Balance is the key to work-life and stress management. Activity, productivity, creativity, and self-motivation should be balanced with quiet soul time, moderate exercise, and regular relaxation time.

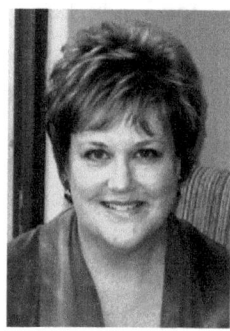

Dr. Arien Van Der Merwe, MBChB (Pretoria) FRIPH (London) FRCAM (Dublin) MISMA (UK) is a medical doctor, author and specialist corporate health & wellness service provider. She presents talks, workshops, seminars and open short courses at the University of Pretoria & at many workplaces in South Africa and abroad. Fields of specialization include workplace wellness, peer/wellness educator training, stress management and natural, integrative medicine. www.HealthStressWellness.com
arienvdm@samedical.co.za

To Err Is Human - To Forgive Is Healthy

Retta Flagg

The mainstay of business is human relationships. The richness of interpersonal relationships in the office creates a complex emotional background that affects all operations of any business. We are all affected by this emotional atmosphere as we do our jobs.

One of the most complicated conundrums for any manager is dealing with a person who feels wounded and who responds by carrying a grudge against a team member or turns against the team's vision or goals. Once their defenses kick in, it creates an emotional pattern that complicates the business pattern. It doesn't matter to them if the result is that someone's feelings are hurt because they were downsized to a lesser job or if someone else gets the cubicle with two square feet less space.

Holding a grudge or feeling betrayed affects your health. The cure for this is forgiveness. Research studies on forgiveness and health show that training in forgiveness or even thinking forgiving thoughts can lower the level of cortisol, blood flow, heart rate, and blood pressure. Yet very few people connect heart disease or memory loss with constantly feeling angry or betrayed. We feel that by holding onto our grudge or by seeking vengeance, we are somehow creating pain for the perceived transgressor. The truth is we are truly hurting ourselves and shortening our life span because of the long term effects of anger on our bodies.

So why do people wind up feeling wounded and betrayed? There are three main areas where basic human needs get betrayed. The most basic need is safety or primary security issues. This is the food and shelter level. Are they getting paid enough to meet basic needs? Is their work area safe? Is the equipment adequate to do the job? Do they feel they are part of the group? Remember that a perceived threat is just as powerful and detrimental to the human mind and psyche as a real one.

The second area is status. This is where we establish our value or worth. It is our vision of who we are and what we contribute. Again, monetary issues affect status issues. Job reviews, job titles, and job descriptions figure into our perceived status. If someone feels that they are doing their part to contribute but the job review doesn't reflect their effort, resentments ensue. I would much rather be called a junior vice president than a supervisor, but if I feel valued for my efforts as a supervisor then I am going to feel fine without a bigger title. It doesn't matter what my title is if I feel undervalued. A violation of status can generate just as much ill will as a major pay cut.

The third area has to do with will. The highest function of will is to feel secure in your identity around people who are different or have different values. If you are on a team and suddenly realize that everyone has different values than you, you might feel betrayed unless your ego can feel secure enough in the situation. People on a production line usually view themselves differently than someone in management, even though they are on the same production team. If the manager and the production line employees have a vision that contains common elements, there is less likely to be friction on issues of betrayal or grudges.

The process of forgiveness happens on more levels than just forgiving the perceived transgressor. While it is important to forgive the event or person that violated a boundary or caused pain, sometimes we stay angry because of our own part in the situation. We might think, "If only I hadn't walked down that dark alley. I wouldn't have gotten mugged." Or maybe, "If only I hadn't told my boss how to fix that problem, then I would have gotten the promotion instead of Joe." We need to forgive ourselves as part of the process. We also need to forgive the social structure that allowed harmful behavior. Maybe only the boss has the access to send through new ideas. Maybe the city could have added more lights to a dark region or had more police patrolling an area. We need to recognize and forgive all levels of feeling betrayed.

We don't forgive easily for several reasons. We don't trust that forgiveness will make a difference in the situation. We fear that letting go of our anger will make the action seem all right. Remember that forgiving does not mean condoning. You don't have to like what happened in order to forgive it, nor do you have to let it happen again. We might hold onto a judgment about the other person or event or even ourselves. Have you ever said, "If only I hadn't been so stupid?" Forgive yourself for a moment of stupidity.

Or we might have a judgment about someone's race or intelligence. Take a look at what judgments might be in the way of forgiveness. We might have expectations; for example, our boss should take care of us—and they are only out for themselves. We might think that we are tough enough to handle any back-alley bully—and they beat us up. If you think you're pretty tough and someone turns out to be tougher, it can be hard to let go of anger.

Forgiveness means letting go. Let go of the need to be right. Is your boss really out for just himself or were you always taught that bosses don't care about their workers? Let go of your need for vengeance. In the long run, you will pay just as dearly for vengeance as the perceived transgressor, regardless of the hurt or injury. Let go of your need to not be wrong. This one is a little trickier to catch and understand, but it's also a very powerful need for the human psyche. On some level, we fear that if we are wrong we will be harmed. This goes back to basic security levels and needing to stay safe. Take a risk and forgive.

To help with the forgiveness process, try the following exercise to jump-start the process.

Forgiveness Technique

- Visualize a sphere of golden light.
- See yourself standing in this sphere of light.
- Now see the person or event that you want to forgive.
- Visualize a bright, white column of light between you and the person or event.
- Recognize this column of light as holding a space of unconditional love.
- Step into the column of light.
- Invite the person or event into the column of light with you.
- Embrace the person or event.
- Visualize yourself merging with the person or event in that moment of unconditional love.

- Make a vowel sound that vibrates your heart to seal the work.

How will you know that you have forgiven someone or something or even yourself? First, you will be able to see that somehow you have gained something from the experience. "I learned not to walk through dark streets alone." "My boss might just be out for his own good, but I am still worthy and have valuable contributions to give." You will know that you have forgiven when you feel grateful on some level for the lesson you learned and not the anger that was sending your blood pressure through the roof.

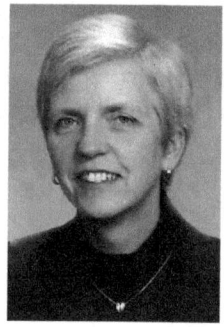

Retta Flagg is the owner of The Healing Touch of Pittsburgh, LLC and president of Integrated Spirit, Inc. through which she teaches advanced massage therapy skills, wellness programs, and self empowerment techniques. From her twenty years of experience in complementary medicine, she has designed practical wellness programs for diverse corporate environments.
retta@thehealingtouch.net
www.thehealingtouch.net

Emotional Wellness: Keeping It Real and Keeping Your Cool When All Around You Others are Losing Theirs

Patrice Rancour, MS, RN, CS

The post-modern world is a stressful place. Expectations are often unrealistic. Roles are multiple. Multi-tasking, whether for better or worse, seems to be a daily fixture of people's lives. And the rapid pace of change—well, there really are no adjectives that fully do that one justice. And through it all, each one of us is striving toward balance and integration as a whole person. What's a body to do?

Right this moment - take a deep breath. Did you just feel that? Your ability to be emotionally healthy hinges upon your self-awareness, your ability to center yourself, and how you manage stress. Let's take a look at each of these concepts in turn.

Self-awareness

The ability to be self-aware requires that we strive to stay in the present moment. Remaining present is hard to do since the relentless chatter of the mind keeps us time-traveling into the past ("wish I hadn't have") or into the future ("wonder what's going to happen next?"). Apart from the enjoyment of memories or the planning so necessary to achieve one's life purpose—more about that shortly—we need to make every effort to stay in the here and now, as this is where our true power lies: the power to create the past we will want to remember, and the power to build the future that makes life worthwhile.

The tricky thing about staying present is that if you are not used to it as a habitual way of living, it will require some energy on your part to practice it. One does this through the use of regular, intentional deep breathing which interrupts that busy "monkey mind" chatter and reminds us, as Ram Dass has observed, that the best way to prepare for the future is to be here now. For example, right now, as you are reading these words, do a body scan, starting at the top of your head, moving down to the tips of your toes. What is happening in your body right now? Are you relaxed?

Tensed? What are the primary feelings you are experiencing? What kinds of thoughts are running through your head? Why are you asking yourself these silly questions?

Centering

You are doing so to gauge how centered you are, and if you are not, to remind yourself to do what you need to do to center yourself. What is entailed in being centered? We have all had experiences of centeredness so we know what this feels like: usually a sense of harmony or peacefulness, a sense of competence and compassion. When we are off-center, we usually feel distressed because we are out of touch with the best we can be. Being present, we recognize and can name what we are experiencing, and do so in a way that is more articulate than merely identifying the experience as "good" or "bad," which is really not so helpful.

Most feelings emanate from a basic five: glad, mad, sad, lonely or afraid. Naming the emotional experience can help us meet an unmet need in ways that work. For example, if I stay present enough to recognize that I am feeling lonely, then I can recognize that calling a supportive friend will meet that need more effectively than eating a quart of ice cream, (which will, by the way, probably not contribute much to my physical wellness, either!).

If I am feeling overwhelmed at work, then having an assertive conversation about my workload with my supervisor will probably help me feel more emotionally centered than spouting off at a co-worker because I am so stressed out. Which leads us to:

Stress Management.

Much of our emotional wellness is really based on that old serenity prayer, which at its essence, is the stress management manifesto:

> *God grant me the serenity to accept the things I cannot change,*
> *The courage to change the things I can,*
> *And the wisdom to know the difference.*

Much of our stress comes from trying to control the things we cannot (everything outside of myself), thereby losing control of the only thing I can (my self). When that happens, we feel emotionally unwell, off-center, and out of balance. Being present helps us to recognize where the source of the stress is coming from, and whether we can change it or not. I can change my stress response by changing my own thoughts, feelings, behaviors and/or choices. I remind myself in an ongoing way that, while I have bodily sensations, I am not my body. While I have thoughts, I am not my thoughts, and while I have feelings, I am not my feelings. This frees me up to dispel counterproductive beliefs, which in turn affect how I feel, which often helps me to make better choices by behaving in ways that are congruent with my life purpose.

For example, being present might help me realize that it isn't my partner who makes me angry; it is me who decides how angry I am going to be, and also how I choose to express that anger. Do I do it in such a way that it solves a problem, or do I do it in such a way that my behavior becomes my very next problem? Staying present helps me turn these emotional boats around sooner so that I can get what I need to feel centered. From a centered place, I can make more reasonable decisions as to how to manage my stress, and thereby restore a sense of balance.

There will be times, however, when the stress originates outside of my self, and I cannot change it. The primary emotionally centered response in that case is one of acceptance. For example, if I get into work late one day because I had to stop for a long train, it does no good to continue to arrive at that train track every morning at the very same time when I know that train is going to be passing. I can accept the fact that I don't control that schedule, and either alter my own route or the time at which I reach that crossing. Much of our suffering is about the drama we create in response to things outside of our control. At any time at all, we are free to release ourselves from the grip of the emotional punishment we impose upon ourselves by remembering to take that deep breath that signals that it is time to relax.

The payoff in doing so is manifold. Relentless uncontrolled stress increases the circulation of stress hormones in the body, such as cortisol. These hormones, while helping us survive in acute crises, were never designed to remain at chronically high blood levels. When that happens, the immune system fails to repair itself and organ systems, like the cardiovascular system, immune system, endocrine system, etc. become exhausted. It then becomes easier to develop diseases of adaptation, such as heart disease, diabetes, or cancer. Emotional wellness is a critical component of health promotion in that when we are feeling centered, our brains release endorphins, which enhance a sense of well being. A molecule called a neuropeptide is responsible for translating our thoughts and feelings into actual physical changes in the body, and vice-versa. The import of this is that while we can make ourselves sick, we also have the power to heal ourselves. If you are feeling anxious or depressed, it is your body's way of communicating to you that something needs your attention. When you attend to it, you are more capable of either changing what needs to be changed, or accepting what can't be changed. And why is this ultimately so important?

Manifesting One's Life Purpose

Because in the end, our physical, mental, emotional, spiritual, and social well-being forms the basis of living a life that makes a contribution—the one we are here to make. We are each hard-wired to do so, and just as we know we are accomplishing what we are meant to, we also know when we are not. When I am living my life's purpose, I feel integrated in all of these areas. Many of us work very hard to remain unconscious—this is a personal choice. When we decide to use the emotional wellness tools of self-awareness, centering, and stress management, we align ourselves with who we truly are and we remain connected to the energy that drives our life purpose.

And it all starts with taking that first deep breath…

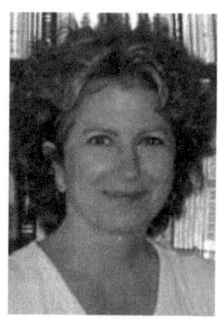

Patrice Rancour, MS,RN,CS, is Prospective Health Care Program Manager for Ohio State University's award-winning Faculty/Staff Wellness Program – osumhcs.com/wellness. She is also in private practice working with people facing life-threatening illnesses. For 35 years, as a mental health clinical nurse specialist, Patrice has been helping people reach their highest level of wellness. A teacher and author, her recent book is Tales from the Pager Chronicles. rancour.1@osu.edu

Loss and the Workplace: What to Do at Work When the World Crashes in Around You

Kirsti A. Dyer, MD, MS

My most recent experiences with loss and the workplace have been with my husband and his workplace. He needed to take time off from work when our youngest was unexpectedly admitted to the NICU (Neonatal Intensive Care Unit) soon after birth. He also needed to take time off with the more anticipated death of his father. For our daughter's hospitalization, he took two weeks off so we could manage with a child in the intensive care unit and a confused toddler at home. Following the death of my father-in-law he took a week off to help my mother-in-law manage with the aftermath. We were lucky because these experiences with loss and the workplace were both short term and did not require extensive leave from work.

In contrast, when my favorite family pet died while I was in medical school and when a dear friend died while in I was in residency, the situation was very different. I did not get to take any days off and would not have even considered requesting one, knowing the time off would not have been granted. Instead I went into work with a grieving heart and did what I needed to make it through the days. I had a different workplace experience once I was a physician in practice. I worked in an office filling in following the sudden, unexpected death of a young physician. There was no bereavement leave given to his staff by the medical organization; they were expected to show up at work, even on the day of the funeral.

When a family emergency occurs or the death of a family member or close relative, workers typically can take a few days to two weeks off for personal or bereavement leave to manage immediate issues surrounding the situation. This leave period is often not enough time to begin to cope with the loss. The worker is expected to return to work while the heart is still feeling and dealing with the loss.

In contrast, when other major losses occur, there may be no time off to cope, such as the diagnosis of a life-threatening medical condition, the breakup of a long-standing relationship, the death of a friend, a miscarriage, or the loss of a cherished pet; these losses do not meet criteria for bereavement leave, but might for personal leave. People are expected to show up at work and keep functioning as though is was business as usual. There is no extra time given to cope with the major life loss.

Grief in the Workplace

These days many people spend more of their waking hours in the workplace than they do at home. Those who work together may become like an extended family. A serious illness or a death in the worker's family affects someone's workplace performance. When someone at work is grieving, the effect on his or her co-workers can be great and can influence the entire workplace. Grief and loss can have a significant impact on the workplace from employees being absent to employees having a compromised ability to think or react.

Grieving Employees at Work

A person who has experienced a loss is likely to still be grieving for quite a while at work. He or she may experience some of the following responses that can affect their work performance:

- Problems concentrating
- Difficulty making decisions
- Disinterest in job-related details
- Frustration
- Irritability
- Tension
- Depression and mood swings
- Marital and family problems

The type of job the person does depends a lot on the impact of grief. In a company that uses production or manufacturing equipment, problems concentrating can affect a one's ability to use equipment, perform intricate operations or monitor product quality. Difficulty focusing by employees, managers and executives may result in losing clients and making poor business decisions that may have a direct negative financial impact on the company. Poor concentration or increased irritability can even affect the grieving person's daily commute and could lead to an accident.

What to Do if You Experience a Loss

When faced with a life challenge or a loss it is helpful to remember the basics. During the first few days following the loss it is important to remember to TAKE CARE of yourself.

This short list provides healthy coping strategies that may help to keep you moving.

Time Needed to Grieve
Avoid Alcohol and other masking medications
Keep to a Routine
Eat a Balanced Diet

Converse with others
Adjust, **A**dapt and Find **A**venues for Coping
Rest and Sleep
Exercise to Reduce Stress

What to do about Work if You Experience a Loss

There are several things that you can do about work once you experience a major loss.

- Ask about the company's policy on taking personal time off or having official bereavement leave.
- Talk with your supervisor or manager about how much time to take off.
- Check about arranging for a temporary adjustment in work hours or workload.
- Consider creating a more flexible schedule.

- Take advantage of Employee Assistance Programs if available. Experienced counselors may be able to help a grieving person come to terms with a loss.

To Work or Not Work – A Difficult Decision

People respond very differently to loss. Some find it difficult to return to work; these people cannot concentrate and are not very productive. Others find it helpful to keep busy; work can help to divert them away from grieving. For others, getting back to standard routines and focusing on their work may be the best way of managing the loss. This was the case with my husband after he lost his father and when our youngest was hospitalized.

Benefits of Returning to Work

Some people find comfort in returning to the work environment. There are several benefits of returning to work:

- Returning to work allows the grieving person to return to a known safe environment with supportive co-workers and colleagues.
- It encourages the person to resume a regular daily routine again, which is one of the recommendations for coping with grief.
- It allows the person to takes their mind off the loss and enables them to feel normal for a while.
- It provides the grieving person with a chance feel productive by finishing work-related tasks. Completing projects may help the grieving person to feel they are still contributing and help increase confidence and raise self-esteem.

What to do if a Co-worker Experiences a Loss

It can be awkward trying to figure out what you can do for a co-worker who is grieving. Many people are uncomfortable with public displays of emotions, yet you still want to somehow acknowledge the loss.

One way of dealing with a co-worker who has recently experienced a loss is to write a note, an email, or send flowers expressing your sympathy rather than sharing the sympathy face-to-face in a conversation at the office. When you see them in the office you can ask, "Did you get my note/flowers?" This simple question gives them a chance to answer more if desired or to not say any more, especially if they are concerned about public displays of grief at work.

When Co-workers Experience a Personal Loss

Here are several additional tips for helping a grieving co-worker.

- Acknowledge the co-worker's grief with a note, flowers or email.
- Let the co-worker know you empathize with the impact of their loss in person or in writing.
- Be aware that people grieve differently. Some people may find work to be a great comfort; others may view work as an unbearable burden.
- Respect the grieving person's desire for privacy. Honor closed doors and silence in conversation.
- Offer specific assistance such as cooking a meal, caring for children or pets, helping with shopping or other errands.
- Remember to include the co-worker in social plans. Let them decide whether to accept or decline the invitation.
- Accept less than their best performance from the co-worker for a while, but expect them to return to their best over time.

Ways of Coping with Downsizing or Restructuring

Another common loss in the workplace is coping with the losses or the aftermath that result from downsizing or restructuring. Some tips for coping with these workplace losses include:

- Acknowledge feelings of anger, betrayal, rejection, disappointment or loss.
- Share these feelings with family, friends, and if appropriate, fellow co-workers.

- Check specific company policies regarding transfers, replacements, and rehiring.
- Seek advice from the company's employee assistance programs or human resources departments if needed.

Suggestions to Help Grieving Employees

Russell Friedman, co-director of the Grief Recovery Institute advocates that companies allow for 10 days of paid bereavement leave. He also suggests that once the person returns to work to allow for "Grief Breaks." By allowing for a short walk outside, visiting the restroom, or talking (a bit) to a co-worker, these short breaks may allow the person to be more productive.

Perhaps we need to be looking at a policy offered in some Japanese companies: *shitsuren kyuka*, a [paid] holiday you take when you feel too devastated to come to the office. *Shitsuren kyuka* is used by employees to recover after the end of a relationship and is offered because "everyone could use a respite after some heartache."

Conclusion

Anyone who has experienced a major loss and tried to keep working through the loss understands how difficult it can be to stay focused and energized while grieving. These are times when just getting out of bed can be a major challenge.

"Getting over" a loss is not like getting over a cold. Some grieving people may never get over their grief. Instead, grief is an emotion that one learns to live with that may get better with time, but also may never truly go away. With time, the intense initial painful emotions lessen to a level that allows the grieving person to function. The grief is no longer a daily all-consuming emotion. Eventually the grieving person learns how to cope with the loss and the grief, integrate the loss into his/her life, adapt to a life forever changed and somehow keep living.

Sources:

Stroeb M, Stroeb W, Shut H. Gender differences in adjustment to bereavement: an empirical and theoretical review. Rev Gen Psychol 5: 62-83.

American Psychological Association. 2004.
Coping with the Death of a Coworker. Available in PDF at: http://apahelpcenter.org/articles/pdf.php?id=120

Hani Y. Sept. 16, 2006. WORKING WITH CARE: Heartbreak heaven for staff. The Japan Times Online. http://search.japantimes.co.jp/cgi-bin/fl20060917x3.html

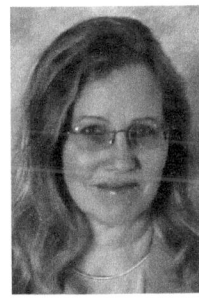

Kirsti A. Dyer, MD, MS, FT, CWS Dr. Kirsti A. Dyer MD, MS, FT, CWS is a respected physician, an expert in life challenges, loss, grief and bereavement, professional health educator, professor, lecturer and author. She received her Medical and Master's Degrees from the University of California, Davis. Dr. Dyer also has expertise in wellness education and health promotion. She teaches college courses in Nutrition and Wellness and a graduate course in Grief, Loss and Bereavement.
www.journeyofhearts.org/cc/cc_dyer.htm

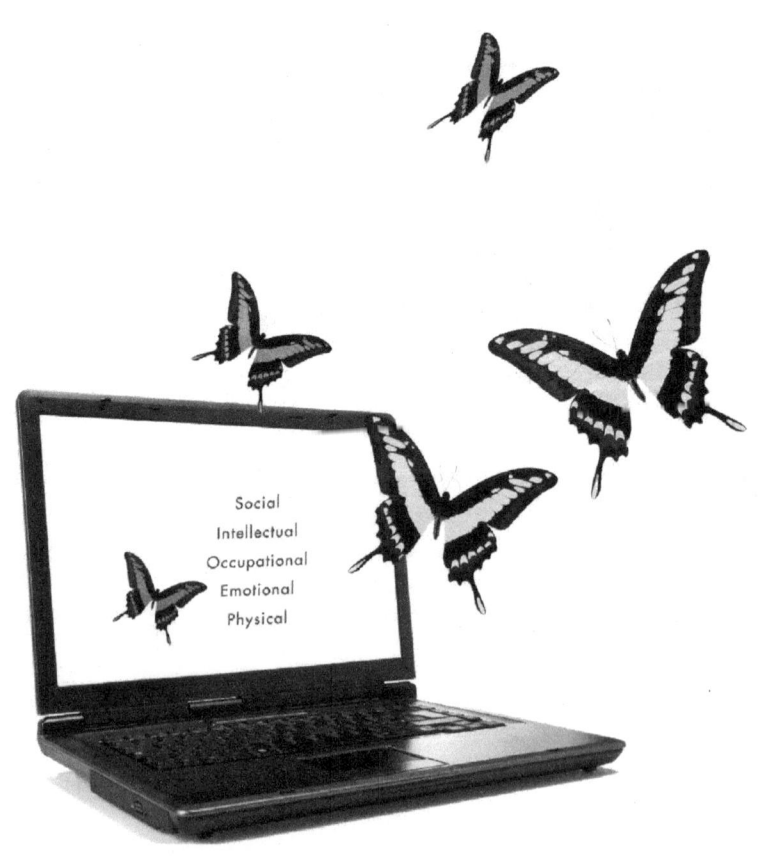

Section 5: Social Wellness

"It is not the strongest of the species that survive, nor the most intelligent, but the one most responsive to change."
~ Charles Darwin

Section 5: Social Wellness

Introduction

Social Wellness is the ability to develop friendships, healthy behaviors, and comfortable interactions with others while working for harmony in personal, professional, community, and world environments. Social wellness can be achieved by establishing a supporting group of social networks through family, friends, group associations, or other meaningful relationships. By strengthening our relationships, we strengthen ourselves to interact positively regardless of the situation or outcome. We begin to feel better about who we are and what we can contribute. With this new resolve, we attract additional experiences and relationships while communicating what we truly desire.

Characteristics of Social Wellness:

- Maintaining positive interactions
- Deriving comfort and ease from work and leisure situations
- Communicating feelings and needs
- Developing and building close friendships and intimacy
- Practicing empathy and effective listening
- Caring for others and allowing others to care for you
- Recognizing the need for leisure and recreation while budgeting time for those activities

The Need for Social Wellness

Did you know that ....

"Organizations today face considerable external and internal volatility. Companies must attract and retain workers whose talents are often in short supply and high demand and who may be unexpectedly wooed away by competitors in 'the war for talent.'

"This kind of volatility can erode social capital, which thrives on stable connections and adherence to the explicit and tacit agreements that bind people to one another and to the organization.

"Volatility may threaten social capital, but high social capital helps organizations successfully weather its ravages. As the experience of [high social capital] firms shows, community membership and commitment to a shared aim are more reliable weapons in the war for talent—especially the war to retain talent—than signing bonuses and the shaky promise of stock-option riches. Similarly, when organizations that undertake necessary changes understand, respect, and take steps to preserve the value of their existing social capital, the changes are likely to go better, because they are accomplished with the support of the members of the organization. In fact, the challenges of hard times or complex change can foster a sense of solidarity in crisis. High social capital helps firms retain their skills and coherence, even when change occurs that would disrupt or dispirit organizations with smaller social capital reserves."

In Good Company, Don Cohen and Laurence Prusak,
Harvard Business School Press, 2001

"Research shows that having ambivalent friendships in your life—relationships where interactions are sometimes supportive and positive and sometimes hostile or negative—can actually cause more stress than relationships that are consistently negative! Additionally, relationship conflict and stress have been shown to have a clear negative impact on health, affecting blood pressure, contributing to heart disease, and correlating with other conditions. That's why it's in your best interest to minimize or eliminate negative relationships in your life."

"The Ways And Hows Of Letting Go Of A Relationship That Stresses You Out",
Elizabeth Scott, M.S.

Social Wellness Experts

Our workplace is made up of diverse teams of people who come together for a common purpose and goal. Rajiv Kumar in "Shape Up the Nation: Using Our Social Networks to Promote Wellness," talks about the team aspect of health and wellness. Read how Shape Up the Nation is creating a healthy workplace with teams whose members reach across the United States. He describes how our social networks influence not only our environment but how we respond in the form of attitude and behavior.

David Lazear gives us a way to get the most creative thinking from everyone on the team next time we have a planning session in "Whole Brain Thinking and Planning."

Devin Hakala quotes in "The Poison of Workplace Gossip," that "Gossip is destructive. In a workplace, gossip destroys trust, morale, and focus." Devin describes gossip personalities as well as gossip-busting ways to remove ourselves from its destruction.

Setting boundaries is a way to alleviate gossip's destructive methods. **Lizzie Linton** in "Boundaries on the Clock: Stories to Live By," gives us true-life examples of boundary setting and how to be your own gatekeeper in workplace situations.

Last, **Mr. Rooney** will show us the value of pets in the workplace in "Being Social and Productive – Pets in the Workplace." Pets add value far beyond being cute and friendly. Productivity increases as well as health and relationships. Learn how to start a pet program in your workplace and a few pointers on how to start off on the right paw.

Let's begin!

Social Wellness

Social Wellness: Personal Assessment

Read the questions and rate yourself from 0 (low level) to 5 (high level) of achievement. Determine the total number for each rating and compare it to the answer key below. This determines where your social wellness stands today. Take the test again in 30 days to check your progress on improving social wellness. Remember, improvement in any area is *positive action in motion*.

1. I see friends or family socially at least one time per week.
   5   4   3   2   1   0

2. I make deliberate time to connect with others via phone, email, snail mail, or face to face.
   5   4   3   2   1   0

3. I'm deliberate about maintaining a positive attitude.
   5   4   3   2   1   0

4. I promote healthy, positive communication with my co-workers.
   5   4   3   2   1   0

5. I'm an active volunteer in my community or church.
   5   4   3   2   1   0

6. I have someone to talk with when I have a problem.
   5   4   3   2   1   0

7. I look for ways to participate in activities that I enjoy.
   5   4   3   2   1   0

8. I have more positive than negative relationships.
   5   4   3   2   1   0

9. I find ways to increase collaborative interaction with work teams and associates.

      5   4   3   2   1   0

10. I'm comfortable forming new friendships and belonging to groups outside of home and office.

      5   4   3   2   1   0

Answer Key: If you answered,

    Mostly 5's you have an excellent level of social wellness. Continue stretching your comfort zone and finding ways to gain greater benefits of being socially fit. Consider teaching others how they can reach their social wellness goals.

    Mostly 4's you have a high level of social wellness. Consider finding innovative ways to make your 4's turn to 5's. This can be fun and exciting.

    Mostly 3's you have a reasonable level of social wellness. With a greater attempt and laser focus, you become the model of what it takes to get where you want to be.

    Mostly 2's you're at a good starting point of social wellness. Allow yourself to begin again, set goals and go for it!

    Mostly 1's it's time for an upgrade. You have what it takes. Make yourself a priority. Wellness is important to thrive and survive in todays fast pace world.

    Mostly 0's choose one area of social wellness to improve upon each month. Seek a buddy to help you find ways to reach your goal, hold you accountable and be your cheerleader. You're worth the investment!

> "We don't accomplish anything in this world alone ... and whatever happens is the result of the whole tapestry of one's life and all the weavings of individual threads from one to another that creates something."
> ~ *Sandra Day O'Conner*

Shape Up The Nation: Using Our Social Networks To Promote Wellness

Rajiv Kumar

Her father died suddenly of a heart attack at age fifty-four. Now here was Susan, in her early forties, rushing to her doctor's office with a terrifying constellation of symptoms: worsening chest pain, chronic fatigue, aches throughout her body.

Susan's doctor ran a standard battery of tests. The initial results came back negative and she exhaled, but she knew that relief would not last long if she continued on her perilous path. Susan's health had spiraled out of control. She found herself succumbing to the temptations and shortcuts that challenge our resolve every day. "My weight," she confided in an email to me, "had skyrocketed to the highest it had ever been."

One year ago, spurred by the memory of her father and alarmed by her physician's warnings, Susan made a resolution to transform her lifestyle and reclaim her health.

Every New Year, millions of Americans like Susan resolve to do the same. Memberships in health clubs soar and diet books fly off the shelves, but the fitness fervor is fleeting as it becomes clear just how difficult it is to fundamentally alter our unhealthy habits, our toxic environment, and most importantly, the way we think. The task is especially daunting, we quickly realize, when we endeavor to accomplish it alone.

It is no secret that we live in a society where personal health is considered a private matter. We rarely discuss our medical problems with anyone other than our doctor. We jump surreptitiously from diet to diet. We wear loose clothes in an attempt to hide our curves and bulges. We join the local fitness center alone, and if we actually show up, we tend to exercise by ourselves. The thought of a co-worker finding out how much we weigh makes us want to crawl under a rock. Many of us go to great lengths to hide our own struggle to lead a healthy lifestyle, embarrassed by what we see as a personal failure. The reality, however, is that we are not alone in this effort. In fact, we are not even in the minority.

Today, two-thirds of all Americans are overweight or obese. Some surveys report that more than seventy-five percent of us do not engage in regular leisure-time physical activity. In other words, unhealthy living is no longer just a personal problem. It is a shared condition that the majority of Americans are battling every day. We are all paddling furiously in the same boat, and unless we realize that we must work together, we will simply find ourselves turning aimlessly in circles.

Susan understood the importance of teamwork, and she vowed not to become another failed New Year's resolution statistic. When she read in her local paper about our online wellness competition designed to promote healthy living through community building, she knew she had found a solution.

As Susan and thousands of other participants across the nation have learned, ours is more than just a weight loss and exercise program. It is a grassroots movement that calls upon Americans of all fitness levels to come together and work together in pursuit of a healthy lifestyle.

The idea behind our program is simple: teamwork and support from our social networks, combined with a dose of friendly competition, can provide a potent prescription for achieving long-lasting behavior change.

A recent Framingham study, written by Dr. Nicholas Christakis at Harvard and published in The New England Journal of Medicine, showed that our health is intricately connected to the health of the people who are important in our lives. If a person gains weight, the study found, his friends and family members are more likely to gain weight. The effect is, surprisingly, stronger on friends than on family, and shockingly, works over a distance of up to 300 miles.

The authors of the study conclude that the reverse effect also holds true. When people lose weight and improve their health, their friends and family benefit as well. A follow-up study found that when individuals quit smoking, the people within their social network were also more likely to do the same. Indeed, this research proves what we already know to be true: that the attitudes and behaviors of the people in our lives have a tremendous influence on our own thoughts and actions.

Excited by the idea of leveraging her social network to help her succeed, and encouraged by her doctor, Susan logged on to our website and took a chance by joining a team of people she had never met from a nearby town.

Over the next four months, Susan and her teammates supported each other as they worked hard to meet their personal fitness goals. Due to conflicting schedules, her team members never met in person. Instead, they communicated online daily, and Susan looked forward to tracking their success and sharing fitness ideas with her newfound health partners on our website.

While she admits hitting plateaus and facing periods of extreme frustration during the three-month program, she reported that the support of her teammates propelled her forward. As their friendships grew stronger, Susan found herself driven to succeed by a desire to make her companions proud.

She went from walking rarely to walking daily. She adopted new eating habits, moving to smaller, well-balanced meals and increasing her consumption of whole grains, fruits, and vegetables. Her new sense of vigor engulfed her whole family, with her children choosing healthier meals and her husband finally joining her on daily walks.

Through her own hard work and determination, motivated by constant encouragement and accountability from her teammates, Susan lost 32 pounds during our program.

Her success—and a growing body of medical research—suggests that one solution to the national obesity epidemic may lie in our ability to bring teams of people together for the common purpose of altering our collective lifestyle.

"The impact of knowing you are part of something greater than yourself has been life changing," said Susan in one of the hundreds of emails we have received from successful participants. "This program hasn't just been about losing the weight as much as it has been about taking back my health and helping others do the same."

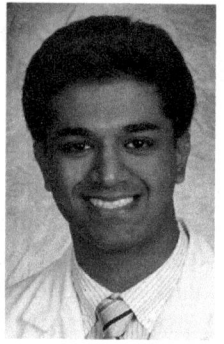 **Rajiv Kumar** is the Co-Founder and Managing Partner of Shape Up The Nation, a team-based employee wellness program. To learn how your company can get involved, please visit www.shapeupthenation.com.

Whole Brain Thinking and Planning

David Lazear

American companies are not noted for listening to and relying on ideas and suggestions from their own people for improving their business. A study of large Japanese companies showed that they ask their employees for suggestions and they typically get an average of 29.5 suggestions per employee of which they accept and implement 75 percent. In the same year as this study, US employees offered 0.14 suggestions of which only 27 percent were implemented. Toyota reports that it typically gets over 2 million suggestions a year from employees and they usually implement 84 percent of them!

Whether you're designing a new strategic plan for an entire company or trying to streamline your group's work process, you need to elicit the best and most creative thinking from yourself and from every member of your team. But it's not as easy as it sounds.

I used to work for a training and consulting company in the Chicago area. When I was first hired by the company to do marketing and sales I was privy to many conversations other employees would have during breaks where they were discussing ideas for improving the company.

Some of these ideas concerned more efficient ways things could be done around the office. Other ideas were related to new ways to sell our training and consulting services. Some were about new products and services we could be offering.

When I was promoted to manager of the marketing and sales department, this source of creative ideas about the company suddenly dried up. I was now part of the elite! Unfortunately, none of these people was ever invited to participate in our company strategic planning sessions. We had cut ourselves off from a flow of fresh perspectives and creative new ideas about our organization.

If we really want to get the best, most creative input from everyone, there are a number of problems we're got to overcome:

Multiple Intelligence

1. Some people are afraid to speak up and share their ideas for fear of ridicule.
2. Some are simply afraid that they can't fully defend their ideas so they keep their mouths shut.
3. Some don't share their ideas because they don't believe they're creative enough.
4. Some don't feel confident at expressing what they're thinking in the formal planning process.

These same people often overflow with creative ideas and suggestions when they're talking with their work mates in the cafeteria or over a drink after work. Every member of your group is a virtual gold mine of ideas if you can find a way to get them to share what they think needs to happen.

Left Brain, Right Brain, Whole Brain and the Planning Process

Probably the most widely known discovery of modern brain research is the finding that our brains have two different ways of processing information: the left and right sides of the brain. Each of these processing modes must be part of the planning process and must be included in the final plan if you want to have everyone on board.

The left side of the brain processes information in a step-by-step manner. It is more analytical, linear, and sequential. It likes facts and figures. It's the professor part of the brain. Your left brain takes center stage when you're balancing your checkbook and trying to figure out what happened to all of your money. The left brain tends to organize new information into categories, patterns, and schemes which it already knows and with which it's familiar.

On the other side, the right brain processes information all-at-once. It's the artistic part of the brain. It likes to see the big picture. It's more emotional, more intuitive. The right brain takes center stage when you're looking at a magazine and you turn the page and there is your ideal vacation spot. The right brain can create leaps in knowing because of its panoramic view. The right brain can invent new ideas that do not fit into any preexisting categories.

Now of course, we each have both of these brains within our one brain. However, one or the other side of the brain tends to dominate depending on the situation we're in. The ideal is to achieve a balance, known as whole brain.

How does this apply to the planning process?

Left brain planners are very organized. They must have a set of logical reasons, even proofs, before taking action. If a right brain planner isn't sure about something, they'll go with what feels right. Left brain planners use facts and figures to illustrate points. Right brain planners use diagrams, flow charts, pictures, colored markers, and models.

Left brain planners are always asking "What's the rationale for this?" "Why are we doing this?" "Give me a logical explanation!" Right brain planners think outside the box or outside of pervasively accepted solutions. At the end of the day the desks of left brain planners are organized – everything's in its place. At the end of the day you can't even see the desks of right brain planners, but they know where everything is.

For the first twenty years of my professional life I worked as the director of research and training for an international organization that was doing rural development in developing countries. When the directors of this organization got together for planning sessions, the leaders always insisted that we make and live by one, two, five, even fifteen year long-range plans. None of these plans worked, but they maintained this was because we weren't trying hard enough.

However, in one planning session I convinced them to switch to the right brain and we started creating a vision for the organization's future. We got some emotion into it. People started dreaming and sharing their dreams. When we had an emotionally charged, shared vision of where we were heading we started cooking! The one, two, five, and fifteen year plans suddenly made sense and started working.

Multiple Intelligence

Obviously, the ideal planning process creates a balance between left and right brain processes. It will be whole brain where left and right are equally involved. This will guarantee that everyone involved in planning process can get their ideas into the stew.

Left Brain, Right Brain, Whole Brain and the Eight Kinds of Smart

In 1983, Harvard psychologist Howard Gardner developed the concept that we have not just one IQ, but multiple intelligences. We're all smart in different ways! Here are the eight intelligences that Gardner discovered:

ImageSmart: *(visual-spatial)* involves such activities as painting, drawing, and sculpture; navigation, mapmaking and architecture, and games such as chess (which requires the ability to visualize objects from different perspectives and angles). The key sensory base of this intelligence is the sense of sight, but also the ability to form images and pictures in the mind.

LogicSmart: *(logical-mathematical)* is most often associated with what we call "scientific thinking." This intelligence involves the capacity to recognize patterns, work with abstract symbols such as numbers and geometric shapes, and to discern relationships and see connections between separate and distinct pieces of information.

BodySmart: *(bodily-kinesthetic)* is the ability to use the body to express emotion (as in dance and body language), to play a game (as in sports), or to create a new product (as in devising an invention).

NatureSmart: *(naturalist)* is related to our recognition, appreciation, and understanding of the natural world around us. It involves species discernment, the ability to recognize and classify flora and fauna, and our knowledge of and communion with the natural world.

SoundSmart: *(musical-rhythmic)* includes the recognition and use of rhythmic and tonal patterns, sensitivity to sounds from the environment, the human voice, and musical instruments. Many of us learned the alphabet through this intelligence and the "A-B-C song."

WordSmart: *(verbal-linguistic)* is responsible for the production of language and all the complex possibilities that follow, including poetry, humor, grammar, metaphors, similes, abstract reasoning, symbolic thinking, and the written word.

PeopleSmart: *(interpersonal)* involves the ability to work cooperatively in a group as well as the ability to communicate verbally and non-verbally with other people.

SelfSmart: *(intrapersonal)* Involves knowledge of the internal aspects of the self such as knowledge of feelings, the range of emotional responses, thinking processes, self-reflection, and a sense of or intuition about spiritual realities. Intrapersonal intelligence allows us to be conscious of our consciousness; that is, to step back from ourselves and watch ourselves as an outside observer does.

One of the things that excites me about the multiple intelligences is that by nature some the intelligences are more right brain; some by nature are more left brain; and others by nature are more whole brain—they integrate the left and the right. What this means is that if you incorporate planning strategies and processes from all eight intelligences into your planning you will automatically be tapping the left, right, and whole brains of everyone involved. The intelligences will do it for you!

"So," you're probably asking, "How do I actually do this?" If you'll go to www.HealthyProfitsBook.com/resources, you'll find a set of **MiQ Planning Strategies** you can incorporate into planning sessions. When you systematically use these strategies, you'll get the best, most creative input from everyone.

You'll notice that on the table, I have divided the intelligences in to three major groupings: the **Object-based Intelligences**, the **Object-free Intelligences**, and the **Personal Intelligences**. Let me say a word about these before turning to how to use the planning strategies.

The <u>**Object-based Intelligences**</u> are **ImageSmart, LogicSmart, BodySmart** and **NatureSmart**. They are triggered by the concrete shapes, patterns, colors, images, designs, and objects in the external world with which we come into contact and interact on a daily basis. These triggering objects include not only the innumerable objects, shapes, patterns, colors, textures, and images we encounter in the world around us but also those objects we see with our mind's eyes through visualization and imagination.

The **Object-free Intelligences** include **SoundSmart** and **WordSmart**. They are triggered by the structures and patterns of particular languages and sounds. The triggers for these intelligences involve an author's or poet's creation via the written word, the evocative power of a musical composition; the sound, pitch, and rhythm of spoken words and their power to inspire, motivate, or move us to action; and the impact of the auditory realm of sound, vibrational patterns, tones, and beats.

The **Personal Intelligences** include **PeopleSmart** and **SelfSmart**. Both involve our own lives as persons—on the one hand, our personhood in relationship with each other, on the other hand, our personhood as solitary individuals. Encounters with our selves and others trigger the personal intelligences.

My suggestion for structuring planning sessions which are guaranteed to get the best thinking, creativity, input from everyone involved is to make sure you include planning strategies from each of these three groupings of strategies. As a *minimum* I recommend that you *always* include at least two strategies from the object-based smarts, and one strategy from each of the object-free and personal smarts. That would give you four new planning strategies to incorporate into your current planning process.

Most important, every person involved gets a chance to contribute his or her best and most creative thinking about what should be done when you use Smart Planning Strategies.

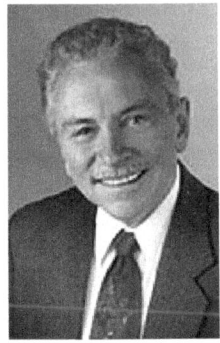

David Lazear is a best-selling author of twelve books on applications of the theory of multiple intelligences for business and education. He has designed and presents Intelligence-Centered Leadership seminars for HR directors and corporate trainers. His training and consulting work shows how to integrate multiple intelligences in the workplace for creating cooperative, effective, and stress free teams and work environments.
www.DavidLazearGroup.com
David@DavidLazearGroup.com

"Intellectuals solve problems, geniuses prevent them."

~ Albert Einstein

The Poison of Workplace Gossip

Devin Hakala, MS, LMFT

Rumors can range from the superficial, "Wow, did you see that fur coat Susie was wearing? I think it's made from actual skunk fur", to the personal, "I think someone said Joe was cheating on his wife with the boss."

The effects of gossip are damaging for several reasons:

- Personal details shared without permission are embarrassing and distracting.
- Rumors are not necessarily 100% true and are often embellished to make them "juicier."
- It is difficult to know where the rumors came from after they have started spreading, and it becomes increasingly challenging for the person who is the subject to set the record straight.
- Employees start questioning which coworkers they can trust and feel comfortable around.
- Privacy might be the best protector for the person gossiped about, who is probably just trying to keep his or her personal life together.

No wonder most people do not want to be the subject of rumor. But some coworkers forget the humiliation and emotional pain caused by gossip and choose to gossip anyway. They aren't all the same either. Here are some easy to identify general types of gossipers to watch for:

The "Caring" Gossiper – This type of gossiper always looks concerned, especially around co-workers who tend to talk freely. Caring people often seem to be trustworthy. Example: "I am worried about Jill. Have you heard anything?"

The Mouth – Everyone knows this person is the center of the rumor-mill. This is the gossiper that other gossipers check in with to hear the latest scoop. This is also the person that people who are struggling—for work or personal reasons—try to stay away from. The Mouth is effective at knowing as many details as possible by digging for dirt on people while recruiting others to dig for more dirt. This gossiper is out in the open, and proud of the role. Example: "Tell me everything you know, because I want to know everything."

The Teeth – These are the minions recruited by The Mouth. For some reason, The Teeth don't possess the necessary experience or skill in rumormongering to become The Mouth. But they are still good at manipulating information out of unsuspecting co-workers. The Teeth take a slightly more subtle approach than The Mouth. Example: "You don't have to tell me if you don't know; I'm just curious. Did Jack move out of his house?"

The Anguished Gossiper – If this type wants information, he or she will try to convince you that gossip is the opposite of their goal. The Anguished Gossiper pulls you in by acting so conflicted you feel the urge to make sure he or she has the complete picture. Example: "Oh, I shouldn't say anything. It's about Hannah. But . . . I don't know. This is terrible because I heard she hasn't dated in months. I should stop. I just don't know. This is killing me. Has anyone said anything at all? I just wish I knew."

The Wet Mop – Picture a mop full of water and mud lifted up and whirled around. A Wet Mop gossiper throws rumors all over the place no matter who's around: co-workers, customers, delivery drivers, basically everyone but the boss. Example: With a patient waiting to be checked in at a hospital clinic, a Wet Mop receptionist says to staff around the reception desk, "I can't believe these doctors. They don't have a clue what they're doing. What, they can't file any forms in the right place? They're all idiots here and I wouldn't trust my health to them anyway." Then, noticing the patient for the first time, "Oh, can I help you?"

Don't talk about a person if you aren't sure if he or she would want the information spread. But what if someone approaches you with inappropriate questions and you're not sure how to handle it? Here are 5 gossip-busters that should help you turn a gossiper away:

1. **The Sincere Approach**: "I think that's something for me and my (family/significant other) to figure out, don't you?"

2. **The Snappy Approach:** If someone mentions something personal about you they heard from someone (which is usually an attempt to confirm or generate a rumor), say something like, "Oooh, let's stay away from rumors today, shall we?"

3. **The Uneasy Distraction:** Once you notice a person is starting an inappropriately private question, dart your eyes back and forth several times between their eyes and their mouth or their ear. Once they ask what you're looking at, say, "Oh, it's nothing." If you are asked, "What is it?" just keep denying it's anything important. The person might feel self-conscious for hours, allowing you to go about your business.

4. **The Openly Deliberate Approach:** Get a thoughtful look on your face, look up and say as if you're thinking out loud, "I am trying to figure out if that's something I want to talk about with you, here at work, in front of all these other people. I'm also wondering why you want to know." Then give the person your full attention again. If he or she keeps at it, say directly to the person: "Now I'm wondering if you are just looking for gossip you can spread to whoever wants to listen."

5. **The Humor-With-An-Edge Approach:** "Do you want me to email you the answer to your question, or should I send a press release to the TV stations in town so everyone knows?" Say this jokingly, and if the person persists, get a little more serious and say, "Oh, you seriously want me to answer that? That is funny."

6. **The Silent Treatment:** You could say nothing at all and just shrug.

The best way to deal with poison is to use the antidote immediately and directly. Using common sense and discretion with your communication can stop the poison of gossip and allows you to earn the respect and thanks of others. If an entire workplace

The Poison of Workplace Gossip

refuses to spread gossip, wellness and health have the opportunity to thrive. Without a universal refusal to spread gossip, a workplace will see an increase in tension and irritability, losing morale and productivity. You can also keep your fight against workplace gossip light-hearted.

You may find that a little appropriate humor may be the best antidote.

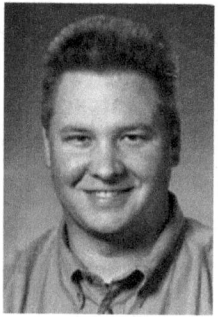

Devin Hakala, MS, LMFT, is a Licensed Marriage and Family Therapist. Devin received his Bachelor's degree from UW-Madison, and his Master's degree from Edgewood College. He is a Clinical Therapist at Franciscan Skemp Healthcare in Wisconsin, where he works with individuals, couples, and families.
www.mentalemotionalhealth.com

Boundaries on the Clock: Stories to Live By

Lizzie Linton

A friend of mine lives in a gated neighborhood. An armed security guard guards my friend's neighborhood. The security guard is the "keeper of the gate." As we drove in one day I asked her, "What do you have in this house?" She returned, "Are you asking me how much I paid for my house?" I laughed, "No, I am wondering what's inside your house that needs to be so heavily guarded. "Oh" she said, "Nothing really, the guard provides me with the security that a burglar or a vandal will be less likely to destroy my personal belongings." She went on, "I really don't have too much of value, but what I have I protect."

Protecting ourselves at work leads to greater health and wellness. It makes for an affirmative attitude and stimulating environment. We are able to sustain our own workload without feeling laden. Relying on ourselves as our own gatekeeper gives us power to grow into wholeness. We protect ourselves by not allowing others to "vandalize" and "steal" our most valued possession: ourselves. We do this by creating order in our work world. Part of building order means creating and maintaining boundaries for ourselves. We need limits that work for us. It's like my friend with her house and property. We need to know what we are protecting. We also need to know when we might be destroying someone else's property.

Separating with Equality: Is it possible?

My mom made it possible. She worked for the post office. We lived in a small town where many of the folks were older, on fixed incomes, and not highly educated. My mother treated everyone who entered her office with care. Because my mom worked alone, the only people who saw her work in action were her customers and myself. My mother cared for her job, her customers, and herself. I knew this because I spent some time resting on the mailbags, watching my mother work. She was the gatekeeper of the post office. Every morning she would put up the mail and ready herself for customers. Some of her customers had limitations and special needs. My mom would accommodate her patrons by helping them fill out paperwork, showing them how to count change, and carrying heavy packages to their cars. This was not an example of trampled-over boundaries or lack of care for herself; she made these choices because she had committed herself to health and wholeness.

Realizing we are all equal is one of the mainstays of helping yourself create and maintain boundaries. When we open the gate and allow someone to come in, we are in control of how and when we perform our duties in our workplace. I watched my mom carefully. Even though she ate her lunch sitting at her desk, she took the time to separate herself from the identity of postmaster. She spent spare time writing and reading. I don't think she realized the importance of her attitude, her helpfulness, and her ability to recognize when something or someone needed more help or more care. It helped my mother live well and gave her a strong feeling of self worth.

What about others?

She thought the sign she hung in the bathroom would do the trick. The goal was to bring some humor into the environment. Work had been stressful for everyone lately and a practical joke felt necessary. No one would know it was she and it would bring a bunch of laughs. She couldn't have been more wrong. The sign hung in the bathroom for several days until a coworker came running into her office breathlessly yelling, "I know you did it! Go take it down." She looked confused. "What?" Her coworker then said, "The sign, someone has complained about the sign." She heard her manager's heals clicking behind them. She ran, took the sign down, and hid it. She came panicked out of the bathroom and was face to face with her boss. Her boss was coming to investigate the complaint. The joke had quickly turned into disaster. One employee on her floor was offended by the "nature" of her bathroom decoration.

Regarding boundaries in the workplace, it's easy to think, "That's my boundary and you need to honor it." This is great start; however, we need to make sure we are returning what we are expecting. Assuring that others respect your boundaries starts with respecting theirs. Boundaries work best when everyone attempts to uphold each other's ideals.

How do I carry my own load?

I worked for a catering company briefly to help out with specific projects. I was the new kid in the work chain, but was told by my supervisor we would all be pretty much doing the same thing. I quickly found out there were exceptions. When we arrived at the work site, there were plenty of items to carry. Some of these items were significantly weighty. One job we had involved a lot of lifting, pulling, tugging, and carrying. The task seemed endless. A little while into the job, I realized one of my fellow coworkers was taking it easy. She did not carry anything heavy. She always needed an "emergency" bathroom break or had to answer an "emergency" phone call. All the while, the rest of us carried all of the heavy items. I asked if she had an illness that would not allow her to lift anything of a certain weight. "No," a fellow coworker told me, "She is just lazy." I asked her why the supervisor continued to let her work if she was not going to do her fair share of the work. I was answered, "Because she is a friend of the boss." Well, that made sense. I watched her as she continued to meander around holding only pots and pans.

With boundaries at work, we have to ask ourselves this question: "Am I carrying my own load?" In addition, we ask: "Am I carrying my load and someone else's?" There may be a time when we choose to help a fellow coworker out and that is fine. However, it should be a choice and not something forced on us. We need honesty if we are working together. We need to be sure, even if we are a "friend of the boss," we are taking on what we are supposed to. We also need to ascertain if we are carrying what is meant for someone else and if so, that we push the responsibility back where it belongs. There are times when we have to be direct and hope the other takes to our suggestions. Is this hard to do? Yes, but you are going to be working anyway. Why not work smarter rather than just harder?

Uh oh, how do I repair it?

The best way to maintain boundaries at work is to establish well thought out limits for your work situations. Knowing that prevention is the preferred method, we sometimes get discouraged when we realize we are "boundary-less." We can return ourselves to a better condition by acting on the following:

- Consider and ask yourself the questions in this chapter
- Start today changing your reality—it's not too late
- Be consistent
- Practice
- Be patient

Finally, know yourself. Socrates said, "Know thyself, the unexamined life cannot succeed." Recognize your limits; the height of your boundary may be a ceiling or two different from others. Make small steps toward creating a healthier working environment. Remaining patient with yourself and practicing consistency will help you to strengthen your abilities as your personal gatekeeper.

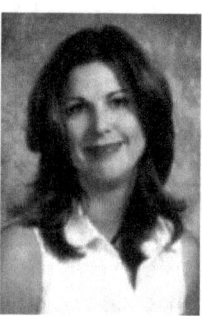

Lizzie Linton is an academic professional currently seeking her masters in her professional field of reading education. She enjoys reading, talking about and teaching reading. The theme of wellness is prominent in her writing. In addition to writing, Lizzie enjoys promoting overall wellness in the lives of those around her.
www.bipolarjouney.com

Being Social and Productive

Mr. Rooney

It's just another day at the office as I begin my security job. I am on constant alert for things that are suspicious like birds, people, or the fallen whole grain Triscuit's from her desk. I am on guard, and lovable. I hear and see with Superman intensity yet find a few moments for a quiet nap. I am Mr. Rooney. I am the Vice-President of Security. I am the lovable "Ruby," "Mister," and all the other interesting names she comes up with including her famous songs. And, I love being in her workplace!

According to a recent survey conducted by The American Pet Products Manufacturers Association (APPMA), nearly one in five companies in the United States allows pets in the workplace.

The survey, which polled working Americans 18 years of age and over, showed some strikingly positive opinions towards pets in the workplace:

According to the survey:

- 55 million Americans believe having pets in the workplace leads to a more creative environment
- 53 million believe having pets in the workplace decreases absenteeism
- 50 million believe having pets in the workplace helps co-workers get along better
- 38 million believe having pets in the workplace creates a more productive work environment
- 32 million believe having pets in the workplace decreases smoking in the workplace
- 37 million believe having pets in the workplace helps improve the relationship between managers and their employees
- And, 46 million people who bring their pets to the workplace work longer hours

Source: APPMA 2006 Survey and
http://www.takeyourdog.com/Get_Involved/win_over_your_boss.php

Being Social and Productive

Pets in the workplace are great for business and the business of its people. They keep us social and productive all at the same time. With that combination, we can put our strengths and talents in the forefront and help our organizations be best in class in their industry.

Since 1999, employees of every size organization have been enjoying "Take Your Dog to Work Day." This annual event celebrates pets in the workplace and encourages adoption from local humane societies, animal shelters, and breed rescue clubs. It supports employers who value pets and gives them a day to promote pet adoptions. Take Your Dog to Work Day started in 1999 with 300 companies. Today, thousands of organizations participate annually. Pet Sitters International (www.petsit.com) created the revolution in 1999. Since then companies such as Google, Advent Software, and Amazon.com have become pet friendly companies. There are other companies following right behind them because of the benefits to the bottom line.

If your company agrees to become pet friendly even just for a day, here are a few pointers from the experts to start off on the right paw.

1. **Do an office check.**
   Check with management and co-workers to see if anyone is allergic, afraid of, or opposed to you bringing your pet to work for this one special day.

2. **Pet proof your workspace.**
   Remove poisonous plants, hide electrical cords and wires, and secure toxic items such as correction fluid, permanent markers, etc. Any office items in question should be placed out of your pet's reach.

3. **Bathe and groom your pet before its office debut.**
   Be sure its shots are up-to-date. If your pet appears sick, don't take it to the office. Pets that are aggressive or overly shy should not accompany you to work. Instead, consider bringing a favorite picture of your friend.

4. **Prepare a pet bag.**
   Include food, treats, bowls, toys, leash, paper towels, clean-up bags, and pet-safe disinfectant (just in case). If you are routinely in and out of your workspace, consider bringing a

portable kennel for your pet's comfort and your peace of mind.

5. **Plan your pet's feeding times carefully.**
   Be sure to choose an appropriate area for your pet to relieve himself afterward.

6. **Avoid forcing co-workers to interact with your pet.**
   Pet lovers will make themselves known. To avoid pet accidents, monitor the quantity of treats your pet is being given. Remember that chocolate, candy, and other people-food should not be shared with pets.

Have an exit strategy.

Should your pet become overly boisterous, agitated, or withdrawn, consider taking him or her home. Never, under any circumstance, leave your pet alone in a vehicle while you work.

Source: http://tinyurl.com/nm2kbk

Knowing the do's and don'ts of workplace pet etiquette keeps us looking and acting like a professional. It showcases us along with our pet as a team of first class collaboration.

At work and home, pets are companions offering genuine affection and unconditional love. National studies have shown the therapeutic effect of animals on humans. Did you know that there are benefits to your social, emotional, and physical health and well being from partnering up with a pet?

- Pets are strong, reliable, non-threatening, and non-judgmental. There is no expectation and no pressure. They are an ever-present accepting companion.

- Pets are patient listeners that won't gossip about your secrets. They're a relaxing break from a hectic life.

- Spending time with your pet can aid in relaxation. This leads to a reduction of stress and anxiety.

Being Social and Productive

- People with pets have a longer life span due to lower blood pressure and lower incident of depression.

- Pets need exercise too. Walking or running with your pet benefits both of you in many physical ways such as lowering stress and cholesterol. Pets help us get in shape and keep us that way.

- Children who read to their pets have an increase in self-esteem and literacy skills. Also, children who own pets tend to be more sociable.

Pets are unpredictable and full of life. In the end, these are two great qualities to have in a friend that keeps us healthy, social, and on the high side of life. Be the catalyst for pets in the workplace at your organization. Partner with your pet to increase corporate social wellness and productivity.

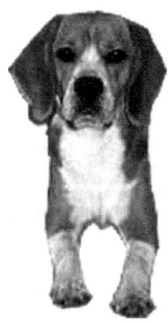

Mr. Rooney is the Vice-President of Security for Sandra Larkin Wellness Strategies, LLC and a Workplace Wellness Consultant. He currently is a published author appearing exclusively in the Healthy Authors newsletter. E-mail Mr. Rooney at MrRooney@YellowDuckPress.com

Read Mr. Rooney's articles at www.yellowduckpress.com/newsroom.htm

Section 6: Putting It All Together

5 Elements of Strategic Wellness

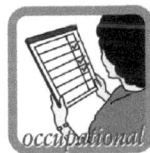
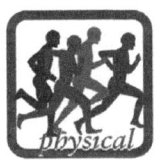

"We cannot seek or attain health, wealth, learning, justice or kindness in general. Action is always specific, concrete, individualized, unique."
~ Benjamin Jowett

Section 6: Putting It All Together

Introduction

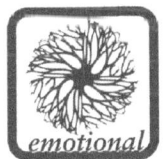
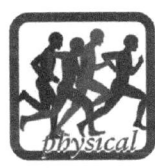
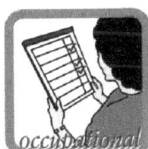

5 Elements of Strategic Wellness

We've heard great advice from wellness experts on how to stay healthy during our working hours. In addition, we've been touched by all aspects of the five elements of strategic wellness. What puts us in a state of flux is that it takes deliberate action, a new set of priorities, a determination to see through the process, and patience to succeed. We put action into the outcome slowly, one day at a time. If we can change one behavior each month for a year, we'll be well on the road to becoming healthy and maintaining the gains made into the future.

So here's a starter. Define a specific behavior to change, one for each month. Use your own "total makeover" as a guide for what to include.

Month 1: Fitness
Month 2: Nutrition
Month 3: Time Management

Putting It All Together

    Month 4: Stress Management
    Month 5: Conflict Resolution
    Month 6: Preventive Screenings
    Month 7: Online Health Risk Assessments
    Month 8: Back Care and Safety
    Month 9: Personal Care
    Month 10: Meditation
    Month 11: Work/Life Balance
    Month 12: Personal Boundary Definition

Today is the right time to "Think about what you can do, rather than what you can't." – Anon.

To show us the results of what this determination looks like, Sharon Frazee and her team at Take Care Health Systems write about a specific program designed and monitored by clinicians entitled *Choose To Lose*. The results are astounding including over 600 pounds of excess weight lost by the participants! Read more of Sharon's case study and be ready to get started making your own choice to lose an unhealthy life style and gain a life of your own design. You can do this!

"In health there is freedom. Health is the first of all liberties."

            ~ Henri Frederic Amiel

Learning by Example: Leveraging Clinicians at the Worksite for Better Health and Wellness

Sharon Glave Frazee, PhD, Ginger M. Barron-Brown, RPH, Sabrina Morgan-Graves, MD, Marcia Hamman, RN, BSN, Myra Wellingham, RN, MHA, and Jeffery Davis, MBA

Healthcare providers who are passionate about their craft produce positive results. These results are even greater when these same clinicians "walk the walk" with their patients, showing, and not just telling them how improve their health and well-being. The truth of this is evident in a weight loss program created and run by a group of dedicated clinicians who operate a workplace primary care and pharmacy at a manufacturing plant in the Southeastern United States.

This program, called Choose to Lose, is not a diet, but a program that focuses on a sustainable lifestyle change for the participants by encouraging participants to:

- Select a low carbohydrate or low calorie diet that will reduce a participant's calorie intake by 500–1000 per day.
- Participate in a walking program that focuses on increasing the number of steps a person takes in a day (tracked with a pedometer) and the amount of time spent walking.
- Participate in a weekly support group that provides a venue for accountability, rewarding and sharing successes, and overcoming the obstacles of losing weight.

As weight loss programs go, the changes are not that unusual. What makes this program unique and uniquely successful, is that the program is run by clinicians—a doctor, a pharmacist, and nurses—who are both group leaders and active participants in the program. The example of trying to live a healthy life, struggling with the same challenges as the patients they serve in navigating food choices, finding time for exercise amid family, work, and social responsibilities, is both powerful and inspiring.

The camaraderie of the group is evident. The experience of a recent meeting held in mid-August 2008 illustrates this. Approximately 30 participants arrive early enough to weigh in before the meeting, which is held in a conference room at the health center. Stickers are awarded to the individuals who have lost weight the previous week. One member, who has already lost 27 pounds in the program, exclaimed, "I worked hard for that sticker this week." As individuals relay their progress, everyone is encouraged: "I have lost 43 total pounds; I have lost 44.5 pounds so far; I lost two pounds this week ..." Even members who have met with setbacks or are on weight loss plateaus are consoled and encouraged to rekindle their efforts. As one participant said, "Even on a weight loss plateau, you feel encouraged; everyone comes to help one another." The four clinicians who developed this program are as active in the discussion as the members—relaying their ups and downs for the week, sharing their food journals, and talking about their goals for the coming week.

These meetings focus on four components that are proven to promote weight loss: Motivation, Education, Accountability, and Laughter. Each clinician takes a turn leading the discussion around each component. For instance, when talking about motivation, the physician in the group talked about her personal goal associated with the program, "To be more physically fit and live to 100," and emphasized the "Top 5 Things" associated with the program:

- **Stay Connected** with the Group (to learn lifestyle and behavioral changes and get encouragement)
- **Take Fish Oil** (to lower cholesterol and promote cardiovascular health)
- **Increase Fiber** (to prevent colon cancer and fiber, when taken with meals, also helps to decrease the systemic uptake of sugars and fats)
- **Exercise** (just move!!!)
- **De-stress** (Stress raises cortisol levels which increases food cravings)

The educational component, delivered at this meeting by one of the nurses, provides written material that is relevant to the current struggles of the group. The educational materials for meetings are needs driven. Each week, the leaders of the program listen to the discussions that take place in the group at the current meeting and determine what information will be helpful for the subsequent meetings. Since many participants had summer vacations and social functions to attend, the education materials for the current week focused on dieting while attending social events, making wise decisions while dining out, and recipes for fast paced lifestyles. The education portion of the program provides practical tidbits to insure dieting success and at many meetings participants commented that they keep a notebook of the materials provided and refer to them frequently.

The accountability component, delivered at this meeting by the pharmacist in the group who has lost 87 pounds, focused on the importance of using a food journal to keep yourself accountable for the choices you make. As one participant said, "If you bite it, you write it." The group leader for this section went through her food journal for the previous week, providing a real and honest portrayal of the struggles associated with a full-time job, raising a family, dining out, social obligations, and the good and poor food choices that can occur in busy lives. The simple honesty of sharing this allowed every member of the group to relate to the struggles of adhering to the lifestyle change of living and eating healthy.

Finally, the laughter portion was delivered by one of the nurses at the workplace primary care clinic. She shared humorous anecdotes concerning weight loss and eating habits. This time allows individuals to laugh at their mistakes, as well as the mistakes others have made, and build greater bonds within the support group. Using laughter as a means to de-stress is integral to program success.

All of these dedicated clinicians encourage the participants to understand that they are not going to be perfect in adhering to their diet. Instead the focus is on the 80/20 rule—making sure that you are sticking with your plan at least 80% of the time. Expecting to be perfect 100% of the time almost guarantees failure. As the physician in the group reminded everyone, there will be good days and bad days as you try to live a healthy lifestyle. Participants are asked to remember the ABCD's for successful weight loss:

A – Attitude, Activity, and Accept Responsibility for your actions
B – Believe you can do it
C – Choose your actions wisely
D – Do it, do it, do it!

As to how well this program works, how can you argue with success and progress? In the six months since the program started (the average participant has been in the program just over 20 weeks), the following outcomes have been reported:

- Total weight loss for the group of 64 ever enrolled participants is 622 pounds (does not include weight loss by clinician-leaders)
- Average weight loss per participant 9.72 pounds or 4.46% of original body weight
- The more actively a person participates in the program, the more successful they are—for people who have attended at least 10 meetings, the average weight loss is 17.84 pounds or 8.63% of original body weight
- For diabetic members (a large percentage), Hemoglobin A1c reduced from an average of 7.2 to 6.06
- LDL down 20 points to an average of 88
- Total cholesterol level average down from over 200 to 174
- Many participants have been able to eliminate or reduce medications

The power of the trusted clinician at the workplace to deliver excellent clinical care has been well known for some time. When asked why this program works for them, the participants said that healthcare professionals both leading and participating in the program has made a huge difference in their success. Now, with programs like Choose to Lose, perhaps more workplaces will start to leverage this power to deliver wellness programs that bring the chance for long, healthy, and happy lives closer to a reality for all of us. This program is having that effect on the participants because of the program's emphasis on education in health and nutrition. These skills give the participants the best opportunity of maintaining a healthy lifestyle for life.

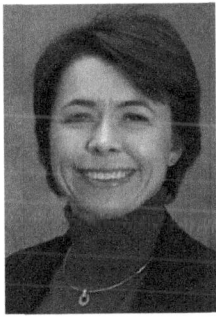

Sharon Glave Frazee, PhD, Ginger M. Barron-Brown, RPH, Sabrina Morgan-Graves, MD, Marcia Hamman, RN, BSN, Myra Wellingham, RN, MHA, and Jeffery Davis, MBA, are employed by Take Care Health Systems. Take Care Health Systems is the nation's leading provider of employer-sponsored health, wellness, fitness and pharmacy programs for large employers.   www.takecarehealth.com

Learn more with audio podcast interviews with the authors: www.HealthyProfitBook.com/podcast

"I don't know what your destiny will be, but one thing I do know: the only ones among you who will be really happy are those who have sought and found how to serve."
~ Albert Schweitzer

Putting It All Together: Whole Person Strategic Wellness

Sandra Larkin

We have the *Personal Desire*   *(The Why)* +
We've Increased *Health Knowledge*   *(The How)* +
Now let's put together an *Action Plan*   *(The When)* =
     Successful Health Journey

Where do you fit into your unique Action Plan?

"Exercise! Eat healthy! Keep a food journal! Yeah, right. I don't have time to take a break at work—how do you expect me to take better care of myself!"

By ignoring our daily health commitments, we put our families at risk in more ways than one: financially, physically, emotionally, and socially. Who's benefiting from our ill health and not so stellar attitude? Aren't we the most important person we need to take care of?

Do you already have a workplace wellness program? Are you hit or miss on planning your wellness journey, having no particular plan? Let's look at how we can combine these two scenarios. The first way is to complement your current workplace wellness program. The second helps you design your personal wellness program when one does not exist at your place of work. Regardless of which way you choose, it's still up to you to take control of your own personal health.

Complement Current Workplace Wellness Program

Take advantage of what your current workplace wellness program has to offer. There are low or no cost ways to maintain health in all five strategic wellness elements. For example, if your wellness program offers these services or programs, here is how they fit into the five strategic elements:

- Walking Program – physical wellness

- Lunch and Learn classes for time management – intellectual wellness
- Community area to take a break – social wellness
- Lunch and Learn class to organize our cubicle or desk – occupational wellness
- Coaching in the workplace – emotional wellness

Designing Your Own Personal Wellness Program

Everyone loves something for nothing, right? It's like finding a golden nugget on a beach full of rocks. We hold up our shiny object and make a proclamation of where and how we found it, and then proceed to the checkout line where we cash in our treasure. In today's economy, we stretch every dollar to meet the needs of our family.

For most wellness professionals, caring for your health and safety is of the utmost importance. So a complimentary offer, (also known as free), helps you on your wellness journey. Wellness professionals would rather meet you on the street healthy than in their office sick with a long road ahead to better health. They provide a "no excuses" way for you to begin a healthy life journey. Finding them is as easy as looking into your local media.

No plan would be complete without appropriate action steps. Here's what to do next:

Personal Wellness Plan Action Steps

1. Begin by listing what your workplace wellness program is offering.
2. Slot each item into one of the five elements of strategic wellness (physical, emotional, intellectual, social, and occupational).
3. Add to your program a variety of what may be missing to accomplish your wellness goals.
4. Find free or complimentary resources to use in your wellness program. Wellness providers are great resources to help you get healthy and maintain your optimal level of health and well-being. During the course of your lifetime, a

variety of wellness providers will be used to address your needs and concerns.

5. Get out your calendar for the month and plan to attend with your family. Make it a family wellness day that includes other activities your family loves.
6. Prioritize your health for the long term by being proactive. Implement, implement, and implement what you have learned.
7. Teach others to do the same! Pass it on!

It's FREE

Where do we find FREE wellness activities to keep healthy and fit?

How do we use these resources to move us to a better place personally and professionally?

Today wellness is all the buzz and all the rage. So it's easy to find resources to help get us started. Here are a few I highly recommend.

Local Hospital Newsletter or Website
These are normally listed as events in their corporate calendars. They range from workshops to seminars with health-care professionals (doctors, nurses, dietitians, former patients, martial arts instructors) leading a group discussion. I have attended great hospital led workshops. Along with dynamic speakers there are also vendors to check out and healthy food.

Local Fitness Facilities (Franchise and Sole Owners)
Look for open houses with a full day of group and personal training. You can benefit from the collective knowledge of the team and get great workout tips in the process. Sometimes these open houses will include other health professionals such as chiropractors, nutritionists, or massage therapists who offer demonstrations and complimentary treatments (reflexology and body work).

Putting It All Together

Health Expos or ANY Expo
Expos usually attract health care professionals and health-related vendors. If you're lucky, the expo coordinator will have mini-seminars during the day. These are a great opportunity to tap into the knowledge of professionals who have your health and safety at the forefront.

Group Health Care Provider Website
Your health care provider may have a wellness portal specifically for your organization. This includes tons of information on getting and staying healthy. Ask your Human Resources department how to access this information from your group health care provider. In addition, some offer free services on-site. Check it out!

Internet Wellness Sites
There are hundreds of websites and blogs specifically about health and productivity. I recommend checking out a handful and then picking a few as favorites. We could spend days choosing "the best one" when a few great ones will do. Pick different sites for your different needs. For example, if you're having relationship issues, choose a site specifically for improving relationships. Or, if you're experiencing a challenge with stress, move to a site dedicated to stress management or one that supports a hobby you LOVE.

Not for Profit Website and Events
Not for profits such as the American Cancer Society list events they will be attending. Take advantage of their superior knowledge of prevention and include it in your wellness journey. Also, they have a wealth of materials such as brochures for you and your organization. There may be an opportunity to have them participate in your organization's wellness fair or wellness workday events.

How do we use these resources to move us to a better place personally and professionally? Great question!

When I worked at my corporate jobs, I planned my month to include one or more of these resources. It became a part of my social calendar which, at times, included my family—events that led all of us to an increased awareness of wellness and safety. YES, it took time to find them. YES, it took time to attend. And, YES, it took time to implement what I learned. But the alternative is what I was trying to avoid ... being sick. It becomes a matter of priorities. In the end, I empowered myself to stay focused and productive, leading me to be a better person, mother, wife, daughter, and employee. Everyone received benefits and it took me out of the 51% zone.

The 51% Productivity Zone

Professionals place high expectations on themselves. Good for the employer. But when we cannot distinguish when we are in the "51% zone," then our health and productivity start to plummet. You are in the 51% zone when you are giving 51% or more of your physical, emotional, social, and intellectual energy to one particular event or period of time. For example, you are professionally devoted to your position and this is great! But when you cannot shut it off long enough to take a break, go to the restroom, take lunch, exercise, or be somewhat social with your co-workers, you've probably crossed the 51% zone. The whopping benefits can be ... drum-roll please .....

- Headaches
- Migraines
- Upset stomach
- Anger or short temper
- Shortness of breath
- Overweight
- Overwhelmed feeling
- Acid reflux
- Bad attitude
- Poor eating habits

Putting It All Together

- Tired
- Achy breaky feeling
- Loss of energy and feeling of importance

Some people are energized by being totally enveloped in the 51% zone. Wonderful! Please make sure you are seeing your physician at least two times per year for a complete checkup. Sometimes the intensity that makes us feel great takes a toll that doesn't show up on the outside but may have silent internal effects you may not be aware of.

Each person's prescription for energy and productivity is different. Here are some suggestions to move yourself away from the 51% zone.

- **Give yourself permission to take a break or eat lunch.** Start by affirming that it's **okay to move away from the desk**. No one will get hurt in the process. My teammates can go on without me for 15 minutes or more. When you come back, look around. Is everything the way you left it? More than likely, yes!
- **Take the steps to move from floor to floor.** This will move you one step closer to any fitness goals you have established. The immediate benefit is that you're burning more calories and getting your circulation moving. Hey, you may even meet some really interesting people that you haven't seen for awhile in the stairwell.
- **Start your own personal walking program even if you need to do it alone**. We had a parking garage on the lot where our building was located. I would walk up the garage levels (creates resistance) and take the garage steps (increases cardio) in 32-degree weather or above. Why 32 degrees and not ALL degrees? Basically, I didn't want to deal with ice (in more ways than one). The benefit is that I lost weight!
- **Graze on healthy alternatives during the day.** Suggestions would be leftover salad, nuts, fruit, or 100 calorie healthy snacks. Your local grocery store has a lot of

healthy offerings. It's a matter of taking the time and discovering what's available.

- **Be in silence.** When it just gets too much, go to a quiet place in your office building or complex or even your car to be in silence. Sometimes we need to quiet all those demands in the form of people and projects to get ourselves in shape for the next round of meetings. Silence helps us sort out the real from the imaginary and helps us take control of our attitude.

These are all suggestions we have heard or read before over and over again. It's time to make the commitment to take control of our daily health. Small changes will not impact you negatively but will allow you to keep in the race longer. They will increase your productivity and health a little more each day and keep you discovering and reaching for Healthy Profits in yourself for the long term.

Sandra

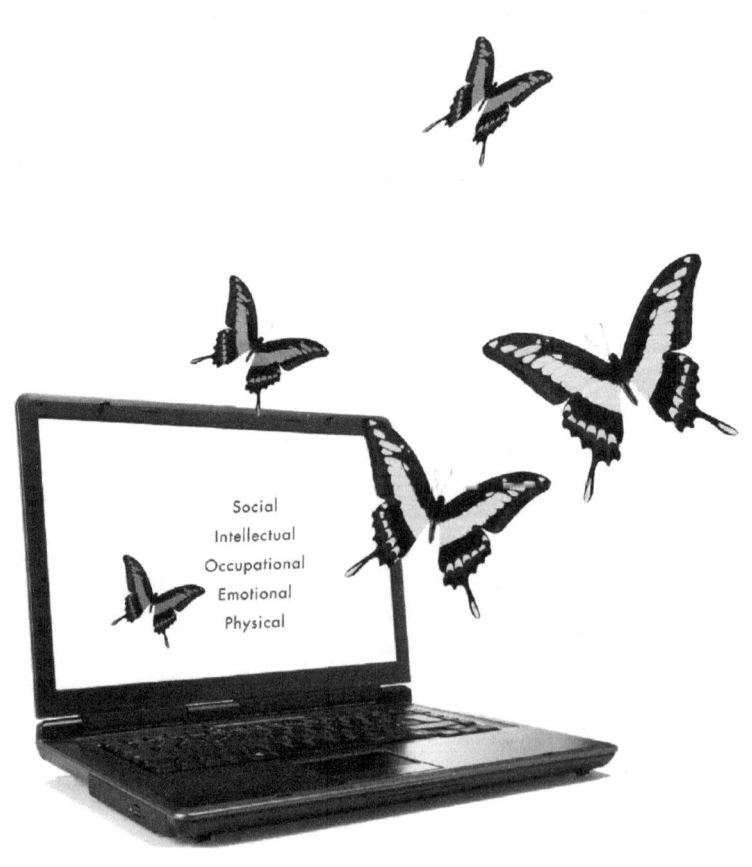

Sandra Larkin Wellness Strategies, LLC

Sandra Larkin is a Certified Wellness Program Manager who designs and develops dynamic wellness programs using the whole person wellness™ approach. Whole person wellness™ centers on developing the employee's total well-being through methods in social, intellectual, emotional, physical and occupational areas.

A strategic wellness program focuses on the continued care and development of the work force while creating valuable feedback for the organization. Management is free to concentrate on business related issues. Sandra provides objective direction, creativity and ideas in planning and delivering your wellness initiatives. Sandra assists in the development of a results-oriented versus activity-centered wellness program.

Certified Wellness Program Management:

- Captures senior level support through strategic methods and vision casting

- Creates an effective cohesive wellness team including responsibility definition

- Collects data to drive health care efforts

- Crafts an operating plan with vision and timelines

- Designs appropriate interventions for a well balanced program including incentives and recognition campaigns

- Structures a supportive environment so that associates feel encouraged and rewarded for a healthy lifestyle

Sandra Larkin Wellness Strategies, LLC

All wellness interventions are customized onsite and results-focused working in conjunction with current organizational wellness solutions. Customized interventions may include training solutions, personal and executive coaching, fitness and nutrition, massage therapy, lunch and learns, personal training, group fitness and much more. Each wellness provider is carefully screened to provide the organization with a secure and qualified wellness provider striving to maximize associate safety and security.

For information about wellness in the workplace, seminars, and training or to book Sandra for your professional speaking event - sandra@sandralarkin.com or www.sandralarkin.com.

Yellow Duck Press

Yellow Duck Press publishes wellness related publications in all media for traditional and web distribution. We work with authors and speakers in the area of wellness and would be pleased to discuss assisting you in developing your content for publication.

Yellow Duck Press Produces e-books, books for print, video/DVD training and information programs, and Audio and Video Podcasts for the web.

Please do not submit any manuscripts or other materials without first contacting us.

Publications@YellowDuckPress.com

Visit YellowDuckPress.com

Contact us for volume discounts on this publication for use in wellness training and promotional programs.

Healthy Profits is also available for sponsored distribution. Contact us for custom logo imprint options and corporate distribution programs.

Additional Healthy Profits materials:
www.HealthyProfitsBook.com/resources

Learn more with audio podcast interviews of the authors:
www.HealthyProfitsBook.com/podcast

More on each author at
www.HealthyProfitsBook.com/authors

http://twitter.com/yellowduckpress